Exercises in ... Manual to

The Skilled Helper
A Problem-Management and Opportunity-Development Approach to Helping

TENTH EDITION

Gerard Egan

Professor Emeritus, Loyola University of Chicago

Prepared by

Gerard Egan

Professor Emeritus, Loyola University of Chicago

Jesse J. Owen

University of Louisville

Robert J. Reese

University of Kentucky

BROOKS/COLE
CENGAGE Learning·

Australia • Brazil • Japan • Korea • Mexico • Singapore • Spain • United Kingdom • United States

ISBN-13: 978-1-285-06753-7
ISBN-10: 1-285-06753-3

Brooks/Cole
20 Davis Drive
Belmont, CA 94002-3098
USA

Cengage Learning is a leading provider of customized learning solutions with office locations around the globe, including Singapore, the United Kingdom, Australia, Mexico, Brazil, and Japan. Locate your local office at: **www.cengage.com/global**

Cengage Learning products are represented in Canada by Nelson Education, Ltd.

To learn more about Brooks/Cole, visit
www.cengage.com/brookscole

Purchase any of our products at your local college store or at our preferred online store
www.cengagebrain.com

Printed in the United States of America
1 2 3 4 5 6 7 16 15 14 13 12

CONTENTS

1006915292

About the Authors

Dr. Egan, Professor Emeritus of Organization Development and Psychology at Loyola University of Chicago, has written over fifteen books. His books in the field of counseling and communication include *The Skilled Helper, Interpersonal Living, People in Systems* (with Michael Cowan), *Talk Works: How to Get More Out of Life Through Better Conversations* (with Andrew Bailey), and *Essentials of Skilled Helping*. He also has a number of other books dealing with business and management, and through these writings, complemented by extensive consulting, he has created a comprehensive and integrated business-based management system focusing on strategy, operations, structure, human resource management, the managerial role itself, and leadership. His *Working on the Shadow Side: A Guide to Positive Behind-the-Scenes Management*, provides a framework for managing such shadow-side complexities as organizational messiness, personalities, social systems, politics, and culture. It also focuses on the messiness and politics of change management. He has consulted, lectured, and given workshops on these topics in Africa, Asia, Australia, Europe, and North and South America. He consults to a variety of companies and institutions worldwide. Dr. Egan sees communication as one of the major enabling skills of life.

Dr. Owen received his PhD in Counseling Psychology from the University of Denver in 2005 and is currently an associate professor in the Department of Education and Counseling Psychology, Counseling, and College Student Personnel at the University of Louisville. He teaches in the American Psychological Association (APA) approved counseling psychology doctoral program and is directly involved with counselor training at the master's and doctoral levels. He is a licensed psychologist and a member of the APA, and has served as an Associate Editor for two APA journals dealing with counseling and psychotherapy (Psychotherapy; Journal of Counseling Psychology). His primary research interest areas are psychotherapy process/outcome with a focus on the cultural dynamics and romantic relationships with an emphasis on interventions for couples. Dr. Owen is the director of the Relationship and Psychotherapy Lab and he has co-authored several publications in top counseling and psychotherapy professional journals.

Dr. Reese received his PhD in Counseling Psychology from Texas A&M University in 2000 and is currently an associate professor in the Department of Educational, School, and Counseling Psychology at the University of Kentucky. He teaches in the American Psychological Association (APA) approved counseling psychology doctoral program and is directly involved with counselor training at the master's and doctoral levels. He is a licensed psychologist and a member of the APA, and has served as Chair of the Promotion of Psychotherapy Science section within Division 17 of APA. His primary research interest areas are psychotherapy process/outcome, psychotherapy training and supervision, and the use of telehealth technologies to increase the availability of mental health services for underserved populations. Dr. Reese has several publications in top counseling and psychotherapy professional journals.

INTRODUCTION TO THE EXERCISE MANUAL
Getting the Most Out of These Exercises

These exercises are meant to help you translate the concepts in *The Skilled Helper* into skills you can use. If you already possess some of the skills, these exercises will help you improve them and integrate them into the helping model.

When it comes to acquiring skills, there is no real substitute for practice. You can practice in three ways—first, by doing these exercises on your own; second, by sharing your responses with your fellow learners; and third, by applying what you learn to your everyday interactions with others in your life outside the classroom. In the following pages you will find a blend of in-class exercises and exercises which focus on your daily life outside the classroom. Classroom activities are important because your co-learners provide opportunities to practice what you are learning and to both give and receive feedback.

A TRAINING PROGRAM FOR HELPERS

As the title *The Skilled Helper* suggests, helpers-to-be need, not just a helping process, but a range of techniques and skills to make the process work. They include basic and advanced communication skills, the ability to establish working relationships with clients, and the skills needed to help clients identify and explore problem situations, identify and explore unused opportunities, set problem-managing and opportunity-developing goals, develop action plans to accomplish these goals, implement plans, and engage in ongoing evaluation of this entire process. These skills are not just bits of helping technology but rather creative and humane ways of interacting collaboratively with clients as they struggle to manage their lives more effectively. The only way to acquire these skills is by learning them experientially, practicing them, and using them until they become second nature.

You are about to embark on a training program in counseling. The following are standard steps you will encounter in such a program. Training programs differ in length and intensity. Therefore, what is written here needs to be adapted to the kind of program in which you are enrolled. Here are the steps in a substantial training program:

1. **Cognitive Understanding**. Develop a cognitive understanding of a particular helping method and the skill of delivering it. You can do this by reading the text and listening to lectures.
2. **Clarification**. Clarify what you have read or heard. This can be done through interactions with classmates and instructor-led questioning and discussion.

The desired outcome of Steps 1 and 2 is *cognitive clarity* with respect to the helping process and the methods and skills needed to make it work.

3. **Modeling**. Watch experienced instructors model the skill or method in question. This can be done "live" or through films and video.
4. **Written Exercises**. Do the exercises in this manual that are related to the skill or method you are learning. The purpose of this is to demonstrate to yourself that you understand the helping method or skill enough to begin to practice it. The exercises in this manual are a way of practicing the skills and methods "in private" before practicing them with your fellow trainees.

The desired outcome of Steps 3 and 4 is *behavioral clarity*.

5. **Practice**. Move into smaller groups to practice the skill or method in question with your fellow trainees.
6. **Feedback**. During these practice sessions, evaluate your own performance and get feedback from a trainer and from your fellow trainees. This feedback serves to confirm what you are doing right and to correct what you are doing wrong. The use of video to provide feedback is essential.

**The desired outcome of Steps 5 and 6 is *initial competence*
in using the helping process and the methods and skills that make it work.**

7. **Evaluating the Learning Experience**. From time to time stop and reflect on the training process itself. Take the opportunity to express how you feel about the learning program and how you feel about your own progress. While Steps 1 through 6 deal with the task of learning the helping model and the methods and skills that make it work, Step 7 deals with developing and maintaining a learning community.

8. **Supervised Practice with Actual Clients**. Finally, when you are ready, apply what you have learned to actual clients under supervision. Supervision is an extremely important part of the learning process.

The desired outcome of Steps 7 and 8 is *initial mastery*.

The program in which you are enrolled may cover only a few of these steps. Comprehensive programs for training professional helpers, however, should eventually include all steps, even though not necessarily in the order presented here. Of course, the best helpers continue to learn throughout their careers—from their own experiences, from the experiences of their colleagues, from reading, from seminars, from formal and informal research, and, perhaps most importantly, from their interactions with their clients. Full mastery, therefore, is a continual journey rather than a destination.

Extensive self-exploration exercises are included in this manual to help you take a good look at your own strengths and weaknesses as a helper. As such, they provide you with the opportunity of applying the helping model to yourself first before trying it out on others. You can use these exercises to confirm strengths that enable you to be with clients effectively and manage weaknesses that would stand in the way of helping clients manage their problem situations.

SHARING YOUR OWN EXPERIENCE:
BENEFITS AND CAUTIONS

A training program is an ideal opportunity not only to learn how to help others but also to improve your own life. It is an opportunity to explore and deal with your own problems and unused life-enhancing opportunities (we all have them). You can do this on your own, of course. But you can also do this when you play the role of client in the training sessions. However, because sharing your own experience in the quasi-public forum of a training group entails some risks, there are laws to protect you. For instance, no one can force you to reveal yourself in public. Instructors have the legal responsibility to see that no one is exposed to harm in the training sessions. Therefore in the following pages such statements as "Share what you have learned about yourself with a learning partner," are suggestions, not commands.

But there is a dilemma here. As an instructor, I have always taken very seriously my moral obligation to the future clients of those in my training groups. The principles are clear. Graduating or certifying incompetent trainees is simply not right. If they don't have the skills, they should not be certified. Furthermore, graduating or certifying students who have serious unmanaged problems of their own is also not right. This is trickier, especially in a highly litigious society. The instructor in your training program should discuss all of these issues with you. You should know both your rights and your moral obligations.

As you will see, the exercises provide many opportunities to share your own experience. You have options. Your can review and deal with what you learn about yourself in private. You can share your experiences with a few people you trust outside the formal training sessions. You can discuss problems and unused opportunities with a counselor. You can be a full member of a training group where participants agree to deal with personal issues openly because both psychological and legal safeguards are in place. Or you can opt for some combination of these strategies.

If you are in a training group where sharing personal issues at the service of personal and professional growth is the norm, consider the following guidelines.

Achieve a Balance Between Comfort and Risk-taking. While sharing information about your personal life is usually challenging and at times uncomfortable, the level of your discomfort should not interfere with your learning or become a problem in its own right. It is hard to learn if you are ill at ease or feel coerced. At the same time the quality of learning improves if trainees contribute something of themselves that is real and substantial.

Deal With Real Issues. Remember that you are in charge of what you reveal about yourself. If the conditions are right, you can use the training process to look at some of the real problems or concerns in your own life, *especially issues that relate to your effectiveness as a helper*. For instance, if you tend to be an impatient person—one who places unreasonable demands on others—you will have to examine and change this behavior if you want to become an effective helper. Or, if you are very nonassertive, this may inhibit you in helping clients challenge themselves. Another reason for using real problems or concerns when you take the role of the client is that it gives you some experience of *being* a client. Then, when you face real clients, you can appreciate some of the misgivings they might have in talking to a relative stranger about the intimate details of their lives. Other things being equal, I would personally prefer going to a helper who has had some kind of personal experience as a client.

Use Role Play as Needed. An alternative to using your real experience is the use of role play. In experiential programs you are going to be asked to act both as helper and as client in practice sessions. In the written exercises in this manual, you are asked at one time or another to play each of these roles. Role playing is not easy. It forces you to get "inside" the clients you are playing and understand their concerns as *they* experience them. This can help you become more empathic. However, an over-reliance on role play is not conducive to learning. It can make skills training look more like a theater class.

Observe Confidentiality. The information that is shared in the training program is not to be discussed outside of the class. Think of this as practice for when you are a counselor and your clients entrust you with their stories of their lives.

GIVING FEEDBACK TO SELF AND OTHERS

If you are working with a learning partner or if you are in an experiential training group, you will be called on to give feedback both to yourself and to your co-learners on how well you are learning and using helping methods and skills. Giving feedback well is an art. Here are some guidelines to help you develop that art.

1. **Keep the goal of feedback in mind.** In giving feedback, always keep the generic goal of feedback in mind: to help your colleagues (or yourself, in the case of self-feedback) become more effective helpers. Improved performance is the desired outcome. Feedback, as we shall see, is at the heart of both training and helping.

2. **Give positive feedback.** Tell your co-learners what they are doing well. This reinforces useful helping behaviors. You might say something like this to a partner whom you have watched helping a client: "You leaned toward him and kept good eye contact even though he became very intense and emotional. Your behavior sent the right 'I'm-still-with-you' message."

3. **Provide corrective feedback.** To learn from our mistakes, we must know what they are. Corrective feedback given in a caring way is a powerful tool for learning. For example: "You seem reluctant to invite your clients to challenge themselves. For instance, Sam [the client] didn't fulfill his contract from the last meeting and you let it go. You fidgeted when he said he didn't get around to it."

4. **Be specific.** General statements like, "I liked your style in helping the client tell her story," or "You could have been more understanding," are not helpful. Change them to specific descriptions such as, "You used a combination of empathy and probes to help her get her story out and to clarify a few points,

but you did not overdo the probes." Or you say to another trainee, "Inviting Carla to explore the kinds of conversations she has with herself was helpful because she came to see how self-defeating they can be."

5. **Focus on behavior rather than traits.** Point out what the trainee helper does or fails to do. Do not focus on traits or use labels such as, "You showed yourself to be a leader," or "You still don't get it." Avoid using negative traits such as "lazy," "a slow learner," "incompetent," "manipulative," and so forth. This is just name calling and creates a negative learning climate in the group.

6. **Indicate the impact of the behavior on the client.** Feedback should help counselors-to-be interact more productively with clients. It helps, then, to indicate the impact of the helper's behavior on the client. "You interrupted the client three times in the space of about two minutes. After the third time, she spoke less intensely and switched to safer topics. She seemed to wander around."

7. **Provide hints for better performance.** Often helpers, once they receive corrective feedback, know how to change their behavior. After all, they are learning how to help in the training program. Sometimes, however, if your fellow trainee agrees with the feedback but does not know how to change his or her behavior, suggestions or hints on how to improve performance are useful. These, too, should be specific and clear. "You are having trouble providing your clients with empathy because you let them talk too long. When they go on and on, they make so many points that you don't know which to respond to. Sometimes it helps to interrupt your clients gently so that you can respond to key messages as they come up."

8. **Be brief.** Feedback that is both specific and brief is most helpful. Long-winded feedback proves to be a waste of time. A helper might need feedback on a number of points. In this case, provide feedback on one or two points. Give further feedback later.

9. **Use dialogue.** Feedback is more effective if it takes place through a dialogue between the giver and receiver—a brief dialogue, of course. This gives the receiver an opportunity to clarify what the feedback giver means and to ask for suggestions if he or she needs them. A dialogue helps the receiver "own" the feedback more fully. Review the principles of good dialogue at the beginning of Chapter 3 in the text.

TRANSFERRING LEARNING FROM THE CLASSROOM TO THE REAL WORLD

The true acquisition of the helping skills is accomplished when they are at your command in everyday living and not just when you practice them in a training program. That is why many exercises are designed to encourage you to take the skills you learn in the classroom into your day-to-day life. The skills you will be learning are not just the skills of helping. Effective interpersonal communication, problem management, and opportunity development are essential elements of a full life.

Chapter 1

INTRODUCTION

Whether you become a professional helper or not, learning the model, methods, and skills of *The Skilled Helper* can help you become more effective in your interactions with both yourself and others in all the social settings of life including family, friendship groups, and work settings. It is important that you understand what helping is all about in order to get the most out of the exercises in this manual.

EXERCISE 1.1: UNDERSTANDING WHAT HELPING IS ALL ABOUT

1. Read Chapter 1 in *The Skilled Helper* dealing with what helping is all about, the goals of helping, and the key ingredients of successful therapy.
2. Picture yourself as a helper talking to a stranger you meet on a bus, train, or plane. When the stranger discovers that you are studying to be a counselor, she (or he) asks you to explain what counseling is all about.
3. On a separate piece of paper write a short paragraph outlining what you would say to the stranger. Include a brief description of what helping is, what its goals are, and some of its key elements *in your own words*. Don't just copy things from the book.
4. Share what you have written with a learning partner. Note the similarities and the differences between your two statements. To what degree do they include the main ideas outlined in the text? In light of this dialogue, how might you modify your statement?

EXERCISE 1.2: UNDERSTANDING WHAT IT MEANS TO BE A CLIENT: SOFT SPOTS IN MY LIFE

Helping is client-focused. Therefore, you need to know what it means to be a client. One way of preparing yourself to understand clients is to review both strengths and soft spots in your life. All of us have strengths, or things we do well, and soft spots, or areas in which we could use some improvement. I might well be a decisive person and that is a strength for me as a helper but, in being decisive, I might push others too hard and that is a soft spot needing improvement. In this case, a strength pushed too hard becomes a soft spot.

Here is a list of some of the kinds of problems, issues, and concerns that trainees have dealt with during training programs. As you read these "soft spots," circle the ones that pertain, at least in part, to yourself. Use the list to stimulate your thinking about the kinds of emotional expressions that might stand in the way of your being the best possible helper.

- I'm shy. My shyness takes the form of being afraid to meet strangers and being afraid to reveal myself to others.
- I'm a fairly compliant person. Others can push me around and get away with it.
- I get angry fairly easily and let my anger spill out on others in irresponsible ways. I think my anger is often linked to not getting my own way.
- I'm a somewhat lazy person. I find it especially difficult to expend the kind of energy necessary to listen to and get involved with others.
- I'm somewhat fearful of persons of the opposite sex. This is especially true if I think they are putting some kind of demand on me for closeness. I get nervous and put them off.
- I'm a rather insensitive person, or so I have been told. I'm a kind of bull-in-the-china-shop type. Not much tact.

1

- I'm overly controlled. I don't let my emotions show very much. Sometimes I don't even want to know what I'm feeling myself.
- I like to control others, but I like to do so in subtle ways. I want to stay in charge of interpersonal relationships at all times.
- I have a strong need to be liked by others. I seldom do anything that might offend others or that others would not approve of. I have a very strong need to be accepted.
- I have few positive feelings about myself. I put myself down in a variety of ways. I get depressed a lot.
- I never stop to examine my values. I think I hold some conflicting values. I'm not even sure why I'm interested in becoming a helper.
- I feel almost compelled to help others. It's part of my religious background. It's as if I didn't even have a choice.
- I'm sensitive and easily hurt. I think I send out messages to others that say "be careful of me."
- I'm overly dependent on others. My self-image depends too much on what others think of me.
- A number of people see me as a "difficult" person. I'm highly individualistic. I'm ready to fight if anyone imposes on my freedom.
- I'm anxious a lot of the time. I'm not even sure why. My palms sweat a lot in interpersonal situations.
- I'm somewhat irresponsible. I take too many risks, especially risks that involve others. I'm very impulsive. That's probably a nice way of saying that I lack self-control.
- I don't examine myself or my behavior very much. I'm usually content with the way things are. I don't expect too much of myself or of others.
- I can be sneaky in my relationships with others. I seduce people in different ways, not necessarily sexual, by my "charm." I get them to do what I want. I'm very good at getting my own way.
- I like the good life. I'm pretty materialistic and I like my own comfort. I don't often go out of my way to meet the needs of others.
- I'm somewhat lonely. I don't think others like me, if they think about me at all. I spend time feeling sorry for myself.
- I'm awkward in social situations. I don't do the right thing at the right time. I don't know what others are feeling when I'm with them and I guess I seem callous.
- Others see me as "out of it" a great deal of the time. I guess I am fairly naive. Others seem to have deeper or more interesting experiences than I do. I think I've grown up too sheltered.
- I'm stingy with both money and time. I don't want to share what I have with others. I'm pretty selfish.
- I'm somewhat of a coward. I sometimes find it hard to stand up for my convictions even when I meet light opposition. It's easy to get me to retreat from my opinions.
- I hate conflict. I'm more or less a peace-at-any-price person. I run when things get heated up.
- I don't like it when others tell me I'm doing something wrong. I usually feel attacked and I fall silent or attack back.

Using this list to "prime the pump," jot down three issues or concerns you have. They don't have to be items on the list. Remember, choose items that might stand in the way of being an effective helper. Try to name issues that have some substance but which you would be willing to discuss in the training group or with a chosen partner.

Issue 1. _____

_____

_____

Issue 2. _____

_____

_____

2

Issue 3. _____

_____

_____

EXERCISE 1.3: REVIEWING MY STRENGTHS

Clients will come to you because they have problems, but they will also come because they want more out of life—that is, they have unused opportunities. But clients, like the rest of us, have strengths, things they do well. The positive psychology movement suggests that the helping professions have spent too much time on clients' problems and soft spots and not enough time on helping them cultivate and use their strengths to manage the problem situations of life. Of course, an overused strength might, in some situations, including helping, turn into a soft spot. I might well be a decisive person and that is a strength for me as a helper but, in being decisive, I might push others too hard and that is a soft spot needing improvement.

1. In this exercise, merely jot down on separate paper, in whatever way they come to you — attitudes, skills, behaviors, and ways of expressing emotions that help you lead a fuller life, that is, your strengths. Here is what one prospective counselor had to say:

- I have lots of friends. I like people. I like being with people.
- Others can count of me.
- I've got a good part-time job; my boss likes the quality of my work.
- I'm fairly smart, but I don't go around telling people about it.
- I am very healthy. I eat right and get the kind of exercise that keeps me healthy.
- My belief in God gives me a center.
- I'm hard working. I get things done.
- I have a mind of my own; I don't give in just to please others.

2. Now review the list you have made of your own strengths. Star three or four items you think will help make you a better helper.
3. Share you list with a learning partner and discuss how the starred strengths might contribute to your being a good helper.
4. Finally, list three strengths you do not currently have but would like to develop. Choose strengths you think will help you become an effective counselor.

Desired strength #1

_____

Desired strength #2

_____

Desired strength #3

_____

EXERCISE 1.4: UNDERSTANDING CLIENTS' EXPECTATIONS, HOPES, & FEARS

Clients come to therapy with different expectations, hopes, and fears which can influence the way in which they engage in the therapy process. One of the initial goals of therapy is to gain an understanding of clients' expectations, hopes, and fears about being in counseling.

1. Imagine that you are going to see a counselor to talk about the issues you chose in Exercise 1.2. List 4 expectations you would have for your counselor. For example, what would you want your counselor to do, or how would you want your counselor to relate to you (e.g., be supportive, give you advice)?

_____

_____

_____

_____

2. Imagine that you are going to see a counselor. List 4 worries or concerns that you might have about being in counseling (e.g., fear of disclosing yourself). Be specific.

_____

_____

_____

_____

3. Broaden your learning by sharing what you have written with a learning partner and discussing the implications for becoming a therapist.

EXERCISE 1.5: TURNING PROBLEMS INTO OPPORTUNITIES

While on the surface the long list of issues or concerns outlined in Exercise 1.2 is a list of problems, it can also be seen as a list of opportunities. Take an item on the list: "I don't like it when others tell me I'm doing something wrong. I usually feel attacked and I fall silent or attack back." Once the trainee recognizes that she reacts poorly to negative or corrective feedback, she has the opportunity of changing her behavior. If she works at it, there will come a time when she will be able to say something like this:

> "When people give me negative or corrective feedback, I use it as an opportunity to learn something about myself. Even when what the other person is saying is unfair, I can listen and learn. And it's an opportunity for self-discipline. I ask questions to get at the heart of what the person is saying. It's not always easy and I don't always succeed, but I keep learning about myself."

Note also that there is a strength hidden in her soft spot: She is not a pushover. She knows how to stand her ground. She has fiber. This strength, when overused becomes problematic.

4

1. Now do the same with the three issues you chose in Exercise 1.2. Take each issue and turn each into an opportunity.
2. Name any strength hidden in each soft spot.

Problem Turned into an Opportunity #1.

_____

_____

_____

Problem Turned into an Opportunity #2.

_____

_____

_____

Problem Turned into an Opportunity #3.

_____

_____

_____

EXERCISE 1.6: USING STRENGTHS TO SPOT UNUSED OPPORTUNITIES

Unused opportunities are as important as problems. This exercise helps you take a look at some unused opportunities in your own life which, if exploited, might help you become a better counselor.

1. Return to Exercise 1.3, which deals with strengths.
2. Read your list and identify two ways you might leverage one or any combination of your strengths into opportunities that would contribute to your being a more effective helper.
3. Share the opportunities you find and talk them through with a learning partner. Discuss the importance of spotting and helping clients spot unused opportunities.

Example. Sonya is a part-time student in a counseling program. She also has a job that consumes 30 hours of her time per week. She reviews her list of strengths and says, "I'm very hard working, both at school and at work. I'm also very careful in how I do my work. However, I don't put the same effort into developing my social life. I could apply these two strengths in developing a fuller social life. After all, helping is about people and I need to get better at people skills." She goes on to search for a second unused opportunity. In talking her unused opportunities through with a learning partner, she comes to realize that she can use the training group as a "lab" for developing a better social life.

5

Unused Opportunity #1.

_____

_____

Unused Opportunity #2.

_____

_____

EXERCISE 1.7: PERSONALIZING THE INGREDIENTS OF SUCCESSFUL THERAPY

It is crucial that you master the behaviors and the values associated with each of the ingredients of successful therapy discussed in Chapter 1 of the text. This exercise is designed to help you relate these ingredients to your own life.

1. Read about each ingredient one at a time, then answer the questions and, if asked to, rate yourself (on a scale of 1-7 with 7 as the highest score) on each. As time permits, discuss what you learn about yourself with a learning partner.

A. Client Focus

If you were a client, why would you think that your therapist should work with you in such a way as to "keep you in the driver's seat" throughout the helping process?

_____

_____

How "client-focused" in the sense outlined in the text are you when others (friends, relatives, strangers, peers) talk with you about their problems? Rate 1-7_____

B. The Therapist. Read in Chapter 1 of _The Skilled Helper_ what Wampold (2011) has to say about effective therapist behaviors. List two behaviors he cites that you think you are already good at and two that you think you need to work on.
Good at:

_____

_____

Need to work on:

_____

_____

C. The Helping Relationship. Successful outcomes in therapy depend a great deal on the quality of the helping relationship or alliance.

1. List two strengths you believe you have in establishing solid relationships with other people.

_____

_____

2. List two areas you need to work on in order to establish and retain good relationships.

_____

_____

3. Discuss with a partner what you need to do to leverage your strengths and attend to your weaknesses.

D. Communication Skills at the Service of Dialogue. Communication skills are relationship-building skills. They are the vehicle through which you do everything in therapy. You can't just "put them on." They must be part of you.

1. Give yourself an overall rating as an interpersonal communicator (1-7) _____
2. Next, find two friends, relatives, or colleagues who know you well and are willing to give you honest feedback on your communication abilities, including both what you do well and what you need to work on. Describe the four elements of effective dialogue outlined in Chapter 3 of the text to them and have them base their feedback on these elements. Summarize the feedback. To what degree does your view of yourself as a communicator coincide with what those giving you feedback have to say?

What I do well.

_____

_____

_____

What I need to work on.

_____

_____

_____

E. Feedback Between Client and Helper. As discussed in Chapter 1 of the text, client feedback—that is, helping clients monitor progress toward goals and the degree to which each therapy session is facilitating (or standing in the way of) that progress—is one of the key ingredients of successful therapy. Feedback from the client lets the helper know if the therapy sessions are on-track or not. Such feedback helps solidify a collaborative working relationship between client and counselor. Because clients are unlikely to offer critical feedback unsolicited, you need to help them do so. This can be done formally using measures to track performance or informally by asking such questions as, "On a scale of 1-7, how effectively have you managed your anger this week?" "How do you like the way we are working on this problem?" "How are things going between us?" Seeking and receiving feedback is an important task not only in helping relationships but in all relationships, and more generally, in life.

1. Rate yourself on how consistently you ask for, receive, follow up on, and benefit from feedback from others. 1-7 _____
2. Rate yourself as a feedback giver. 1-7 _____
3. Think of a time in your life when you asked for feedback from someone, received it, and benefitted from it. What difference did it make in your life? Briefly describe how you asked for feedback and how it was helpful.

7

Example: After a presentation, Ramzi, a young researcher in social psychology, asked several colleagues how the presentation went. Just about everybody, in one way or another, said, "It went fine." However, one colleague said that she noticed that he had gone through the presentation hurriedly and made little eye contact with the audience. She also noticed that some members of the audience drifted off. After being initially defensive, Ramzi quickly recognized that this was true and acknowledged how nervous he was. The feedback provided two insights. First, he was overly concerned about what his colleagues thought of him. And, second, he realized that his poor presentation style meant that he did not get the two main findings of his research across. He did not allow the research to speak for itself.

What role, if any, does giving feedback to others play in your life?

_____

_____

What value, if any, would increasing feedback to others add to your life?

_____

_____

What role does asking for feedback play in your life?

_____

_____

How might increasing requests for feedback add value to your life?

_____

_____

4. If you were a client, what kind of feedback would you like to give and receive in order to get the most out of the therapy sessions? What should you do? What should the helper do? Jot down some ideas and then discuss them with a learning partner.

_____

_____

_____

F. The Model, Method, or Approach to Treatment. You can probably name a number of different kinds of therapy: cognitive therapy, behavioral therapy, emotion-focused therapy, psychoanalysis—and the list goes on and on. Read the "Treatment Model and Its Methods and Techniques" section in Chapter 1 of the text.

8

1. Someone says to you, "There are dozens of approaches to therapy. And so they must all be meaningless! What if physicists went about their research that way?" How would you respond? Jot down a few ideas that would be included in your response.

_____

_____

_____

2. See yourself in the role of the client. From that perspective name some things that should be common to all forms of therapy. Compare your list with the list of a learning partner.

_____

_____

_____

G. The Standard Problem-Management Process. Problem management is at the heart of just about every approach to helping. Therefore, it is one of the key ingredients of successful therapy. Read the section on problem management in Chapter 1 (and, if you want, elaborate on it by reading Chapter 8 of the text).

1. Rate yourself: To what degree is this problem-management process part and parcel of your everyday life? 1-7 _____

2. Name some things you could do to embed this process in your everyday life.

_____

_____

_____

3. Let's say that you describe the standard problem-management process to someone you know and the person says, "Oh, I know that! You're not telling me anything new." How might you respond creatively to that person? Jot down a few ideas.

_____

_____

_____

H. Decision Making. Read the section on decision making in Chapter 1 of the text.

1. Rate yourself as a decision maker (1-7). _____

9

2. Why can therapy be called an exercise in decision making? Jot down a few ideas.

_____

_____

_____

3. Describe a lousy decision you have made. What made it lousy?

_____

_____

_____

4. Describe a good decision you have made. What made it good?

_____

_____

_____

5. What is your decision making culture or style? How do you go about making decisions? What can you do to improve the effectiveness of your decision making style?

_____

_____

_____

_____

I. The Beliefs, Values, Norms, Ethics, and Morality Factors of Life. Look at the world from the point of view of this set of factors. They make the world rich, diverse, antagonistic, livable, dangerous, engrossing, and daunting—all at the same time. They have a similar impact on the lives of clients. They insinuate themselves into every aspect of the helping process well beyond the statements found in the APA writings on ethics. They present one of the most formidable challenges for helpers. Read the pertinent section in the text first.

1. How would you respond if someone were to say to you, "There's nothing scientific about that set of factors"? Jot down a few ideas.

_____

_____

_____

2. What do you do when you meet someone (eventually, a client) whose beliefs, values, norms, ethics, and morality are significantly different from yours, in whole or in part? Jot down a few ideas.

_____

_____

_____

3. Helping involves a great deal of decision making on the part of both clients and counselors. How does the beliefs, values, norms, ethics, and morality set of factors relate to decision making?

_____

_____

_____

11

Chapter 2

THE HELPING RELATIONSHIP:
VALUES IN ACTION

It is important for you to take initiative in determining the kinds of values you want to pervade the helping process and relationship. Too often such values are taken for granted. The position taken in Chapter Two of *The Skilled Helper* is that values should provide guidance for everything you do in your interactions with clients.

As indicated in the text, the values that should permeate your helping relationships and practice must be owned by you. Learning about values from others is very important, but mindless adoption of the values promoted by the helping professions without reflection inhibits your owning and practicing them. You need to wrestle with your values a bit to make them your own. In addition, your values must actually make a difference in your interactions with clients. That is, they must be values-in-use and not merely espoused values. Your clients will get a feeling for your values, not from what you say, but from what you do.

EXERCISE 2.1: KEY MESSAGES FOR ME

There's a lot to absorb in Chapter 2, especially if you are training to become a therapist. It is easy to get buried in the avalanche of messages cascading from theory and research in the helping professions. One of your tasks is to organize and simplify all of this at the service of your clients.

1. Therefore, read the chapter and make jottings, but then write down four messages or "takeaways" that strike *you* as key. These are messages that you can embed within yourself and take with you into your encounters with clients.

Message #1:

_____

_____

_____

Message #2:

_____

_____

_____

Message #3:

_____

_____

_____

12

Message #4:

_____

_____

_____

2. Share your takeaways with a learning partner. What was the same? What was different?

EXERCISE 2.2: "IF I WERE A CLIENT . . ."

1. With a learning partner, watch a video or movie segment of a counseling session. For instance, one possibility that you will find on YouTube is a video of the late Albert Ellis counseling the client, Gloria. Carefully observe the counselor and how he/she works with the client. Imagine you are the client depicted and answer the following questions. Jot down words, phrases, or simple sentences in response.

What did you like about the counselor? What did he/she do well?

_____

_____

_____

_____

_____

What would you want to change about the counselor?

_____

_____

_____

_____

If you were the client, how would you have interacted with the counselor?

_____

_____

_____

13

_____

_____

2. Share your thoughts with your learning partner. Discuss both the similarities and the differences between your responses.

EXERCISE 2.3: BUILDING AND MAINTAINING RELATIONSHIPS

It goes without saying that the relationship between helper and client is important. Your job is to build the kind of relationship with each client that contributes to problem-managing and opportunity-developing outcomes. This exercise asks you to look at your strengths and weaknesses in establishing and maintaining relationships in your everyday life.

1. Identify your best and your worst (or at least one that has been difficult) relationships. Briefly describe your relationship with each person.

Best relationship: _____

_____

_____

Worst/Difficult relationship: _____

_____

_____

2. What did you do best in establishing and trying to maintain these relationships?

Best relationship: _____

_____

_____

Worst/Difficult relationship: _____

_____

_____

14

3. What mistakes have you made in each relationship?

Best relationship: _____

_____

_____

Worst/Difficult relationship: _____

_____

_____

4. What have you done to recover from mistakes in each relationship? How are these different in each relationship?

Best relationship: _____

_____

_____

Worst/Difficult relationship: _____

_____

_____

5. What do you need to do to become better at establishing and maintaining good working relationships with others?

Best relationship: _____

_____

_____

Worst/Difficult relationship: _____

_____

_____

6. Discuss your responses with a learning partner.

EXERCISE 2.4: YOUR PRELIMINARY STATEMENT OF VALUES

1. On a separate piece of paper write a preliminary statement of values based on what you learned from the previous exercise. Write it in such a way that you could give it to a client, saying, "These are the values that underlie and permeate the helping process."

2. The values we have as helpers are certainly shaped by our education and training, but they are also shaped by other things such as our families, religion, culture, society, and other life experiences. Consider and briefly note a couple of experiences and sociocultural factors that have influenced your statement of values.

3. Share your statement with a learning partner. Note both the similarities and the differences. In the light of your statements, tell each other what your hopes and fears would be were you to be your learning partner's client.

4. Finally, read Chapter 2 in *The Skilled Helper*. That chapter deals with the importance of the relationship between the client and helper together with a discussion of values that should permeate that relationship. In the light of what you learn, revise your value statement and share it with your learning partner.

EXERCISE 2.5: FIVE KEY VALUES—A SELF-ASSESSMENT

The five values highlighted in Chapter 2 are respect, empathy, proactive appreciation of diversity, client empowerment (together with self-responsibility), and a bias toward action. After reading the section in the book on each value, make a personal statement as to the place this value presently has in your life. How do you put each value into action in your life? Are there times when you have put any of them "on hold"? If so, what was going in your life to cause you to deviate from any given value?

Respect:

_____

_____

_____

Empathy:

_____

_____

_____

Proactive Appreciation of Diversity:

_____

_____

_____

Client Empowerment and Self-Responsibility

_____

_____

_____

A Bias Toward Action

_____

_____

_____

EXERCISE 2.6: WORKING WITH DIVERSITY—A SELF-ASSESSMENT

As a helper, you will meet clients who differ from you in many ways: abilities, accent, age, attractiveness, color, developmental stage, disabilities, economic status, education, ethnicity, fitness, gender, group culture, health, national origin, occupation, personal culture, personality variables, politics, problem type, religion, sexual orientation, social status, and values—to name some of the major categories. These differences come with inherent advantages and disadvantages. Your ability to work with clients who are different, and sometimes quite different, from you is one of the major requirements for being an effective helper. On a scale from 1-7 (with 7 a very high score) rate yourself on the following statements. Try to be as honest as possible in your self-appraisal. We all have room for growth when it comes to being aware and positively embracing diversity. Just look around the world.

- _____ I enjoy meeting and interacting with people who are different from me.
- _____ I would not like to live (don't like living) in a homogeneous culture.
- _____ Even when my initial reactions to people are negative, I try to understand rather than judge them.
- _____ I fully understand that people (including myself) are not perfect and I make reasonable allowances for this.
- _____ I probably have blind spots when it comes to the way I treat people, but I'd like to know what they are so that I can deal with them.
- _____ I see culture as a two-way street: I want to understand and respect the cultural differences of others, but I also expect them to do the same for me.
- _____ I realize that my understanding of other people's cultures will always be partial and fallible.
- _____ I want to understand others in the key diversity and cultural contexts of their lives.
- _____ Because of the richness of human diversity, when I meet and deal with others I am always a learner.
- _____ I think that it is important for me to understand whatever diversity and cultural biases (such as racism, anti-Arabism, anti-Semitism, and the like) I have and to deal with them.
- _____ Although I realize that differences can be a cause of conflict, I believe that differences can also be a source of human enrichment.

Consider your high scores and your low scores. Share key insights about yourself with a friend or learning partner.

17

PART II
THE THERAPEUTIC DIALOGUE:
COMMUNICATION AND RELATIONSHIP-BUILDING SKILLS

Chapter 3

EMPATHIC PRESENCE: TUNING IN AND LISTENING

Part II of *The Skilled Helper* deals with the communication skills needed to engage clients in a therapeutic dialogue. The quality of the dialogue affects everything in the problem-management process. This chapter has three parts: the importance of dialogue, the skill of attending or tuning in, and the skill of active listening.

THE IMPORTANCE OF DIALOGUE

As useful as dialogue might be in human communication, it is not that common—at least in its fullness. Helpers need to become skilled in dialogue themselves and in helping clients engage in dialogue.

EXERCISE 3.1: UNDERSTANDING AND PERSONALIZING THE FOUR REQUIREMENTS OF TRUE DIALOGUE

1. Read the section in Chapter 3 that describes the requirements of a true dialogue—turn taking, connecting, mutual influencing, and co-creating outcomes.
2. Think of an important and, if possible, relatively recent conversation that went poorly.
3. Which elements of dialogue were missing or done poorly and therefore might have contributed to the conversation's poor outcome?

_____

_____

_____

_____

4. Next, think of an important conversation that went well.
5. Which elements of effective dialogue might have contributed to the success of this conversation?

_____

_____

_____

_____

6. Share your findings with a learning partner.
7. Rate yourself (1-7) on your competence in engaging in dialogue and generally conducting serious conversations in the spirit of dialogue. _____

18

EXERCISE 3.2: DIALOGUE IN EVERYDAY LIFE

Not all conversations need to be true dialogues. However, most conversations would probably be more productive if they were conducted in the *spirit* of dialogue. Often enough, dialogue in its fullest sense would make a big difference to the outcome of the conversation.

1. In this exercise, have a conversation with your learning partner. Choose any topic that has some substance and is agreeable to both of you. Talk for about 10 minutes. Make a video of the session.
2. After ten minutes play the video and debrief the conversation in the light of the requirements of dialogue.

The subject of the conversation. What was the conversation about? What substance did it have? Did it have enough substance to warrant a serious dialogue?

_____

_____

_____

In what ways did it live up to the requirements of dialogue?

_____

_____

_____

In what way did it fail to live up to these requirements?

_____

_____

_____

3. Continue the conversation for another 10 minutes. Video it. Make every effort to make it a dialogue. After 10 more minutes stop and review the video with your partner again. Discuss what progress was made. What positive outcome, if any, did the two of you co-create through the conversation? Determine what it would take to make dialogue or the spirit of dialogue second nature to your communication style.

ATTENDING: VISIBLY TUNING IN

Your posture, gestures, facial expressions, and voice all send nonverbal messages to your clients. The purpose of the exercises in this section is to make you aware of the different kinds of nonverbal messages you send to clients through such things as body posture, facial expressions, and voice quality, and how to use nonverbal behavior to make contact and communicate with them. It is important that what you say verbally is reinforced rather than muddled or contradicted by your nonverbal messages. There are two important messages about nonverbal behavior in this chapter. First, use your posture, gestures, facial expressions, and voice to *send messages* you want to clients to hear, such as, "I'm listening to you very carefully" or "I know what you're saying is difficult for you, but I'm with you." Second, become aware of the messages your clients are sending to you through their nonverbal behaviors. Learn how to understand them without over-interpreting them.

19

EXERCISE 3.3: WATCHING YOURSELF IN ACTION

After reading the section on visibly tuning in, replay the videos that you made for Exercise 3.2. Debrief them with your learning partner. How effectively did you tune in? How did your nonverbal behavior contribute to or detract from the dialogue? How would you describe your psychological presence? Provide constructive feedback to each other.

EXERCISE 3.4: VISIBLY TUNING IN TO OTHERS IN EVERYDAY CONVERSATIONS

This is another exercise for you to do outside the training group in your everyday life. Observe the way you attend to others for a week or two — at home, with friends, at school, at work. Observe the quality of your presence to others when you engage in conversations with them. Of course, even being asked to "watch yourself" will induce changes in your behavior; you will probably tune in more effectively than you ordinarily do. The purpose of this exercise is to sensitize you to attending behaviors in general and to get some idea of what your day-to-day attending style looks like. First, though, read about the skills of tuning in or attending in *The Skilled Helper*.

1. Rate yourself right now on a scale from 1-7 on how effectively you think you pay attention or tune in to others—your physical and psychological presence—in your everyday conversations. _____

2. Without becoming preoccupied with every little behavior, watch yourself for a week as you tune in (or fail to tune in) to others in your everyday conversations—that is, how you are present to those with whom you interact.

3. What are you like when you are with others, especially in serious situations? What do you do well? What do you fail to do?

4. After the week has passed, re-rate yourself _____

5. What have you learned about your conversation style through this exercise? Read the following example, and then write your own summary of what you have learned about yourself.

Example. Here is what one trainee wrote: "I found myself tuning in better to people I like. When I was with someone neutral, I found that my eyes and my mind would wander. I also found that it's easier for me to tune in to others when I'm rested and alert. When I'm physically uncomfortable or tired, I don't put in much effort to tune in. I was unpleasantly surprised to find out how easily distracted I am. Often I was there, but I really wasn't there. However, simply by paying attention to tuning in skills, I was with others more fully, even with neutral people. I'm just beginning to become aware of the quality of my psychological presence in conversations."

6. Describe your style of interacting with others.

_____

_____

_____

_____

_____

7. Name two things you could do to improve how you are present to others.

_____

_____

_____

EXERCISE 3.5: OBSERVING AND GIVING FEEDBACK ON QUALITY OF PRESENCE

In the training sessions, make sure that your nonverbal behavior is helping you work effectively with others and sending the messages you want to send. This exercise, then, pertains to the entire length of the training program. You are asked to give ongoing feedback both to yourself and to the other members of the training group on the quality of your presence to one another as you interact, learn, and practice helping skills. Recall especially the basic elements of visibly tuning in summarized by the acronym *SOLER*. Here is a checklist to help you provide that feedback to yourself and your fellow helpers. Review the criteria for giving useful feedback found in the Introduction to the Exercises.

- How effectively are you using postural cues to indicate your willingness to work with the client?
- In what ways do you distract clients and observers from the task at hand, for instance, by fidgeting?
- How flexible are you when engaging in SOLER behaviors? To what degree do these behaviors help you be with the client?
- How natural is it for you to tune in to the client? What indications are there that you are not being yourself?
- To what degree is your psychological presence reflected in your physical presence?
- What are you like when you miss the mark?
- What are you like when you are at your best?

The ongoing question is: What do I have to do to become more effectively present to my clients both physically and psychologically? Your posture and nonverbal behavior are an important part of your presence, but there is more to presence than *SOLER* activities. There are the values and spirit you bring to your encounters with your clients.

ACTIVE LISTENING

Read the sections on active listening in Chapter 3 of *The Skilled Helper*. Effective helpers are active listeners. When you listen to clients, you listen to their stories. Some of the elements of these stories are:

- their *experiences*, what they see as happening to them;
- their *behaviors*, what they do or fail to do;
- their *affect*, the feelings and emotions that arise from their experiences and behaviors;
- the *core messages* in their stories;
- their *points of view* expressed in their stories, including the reasons for their points of view and the implications for holding any given point of view;
- the *decisions* they are making, together with the reasons for and implications or possible consequences of those decisions;
- their *intentions and proposals*, that is, the goals they want to pursue and the actions they intend to engage in;
- the *wider context* of their stories, points of view, decisions, and intentions;
- any *particular "slant"* they tend to give to any or all of the above.

Helpers listen carefully in order to respond with both understanding and at times, as we shall see later, some sort of invitation to self-challenge. Let's start by having you listen to yourself.

EXERCISE 3.6: LISTENING TO YOURSELF AS A PROBLEM SOLVER

In this exercise you are asked to "listen to yourself" in retrospect as you worked through some important problem situation or spotted and developed some unused opportunity. Retell the story to yourself in summary form.

Example. Here is Acantha's story in summary form. "What I have to say is retrospective. I don't believe I was thinking this clearly back then. I got drunk during a football game and don't recall clearly what happened afterwards. I woke up in a guy's room. I knew I had been violated. I had no intention of having sex. At this point I became very aware of what I was doing. My intention that day was to relax and have fun. My assumption was that no one I was with had any ulterior motives. In one way I was not thinking straight. I should never have drunk too much, but at the time I did not say that to myself. I never made a decision to throw caution to the wind, but I did by letting others help me get drunk. My decision making abilities were lost. As soon as I woke up I began gathering my resources. I went for a long walk and thought things through. I decided not to confront anyone except myself. Although I hoped that I would not be pregnant, I began thinking how I would handle a pregnancy. Finally, I thought I needed to talk all of this through with a friend or, perhaps better, an objective counselor." Now jot down a few highlights regarding how you manage your problem situation.

1. Debrief Acantha's story by answering the following questions.

What was the issue?

_____

_____

What were her key experiences, that is, what happened to her?

_____

_____

What points of view of hers were involved?

_____

_____

What decisions did she make?

_____

_____

What emotions did she experience and express?

_____

_____

What did she do to cope with the problem or develop the opportunity?

_____

_____

2. Provide a case from your own life.
3. Debrief by answering the above questions.

EXERCISE 3.7: LISTENING TO MYSELF AS A PERSON WITH FEELINGS AND EMOTIONS

Since emotions are strong motivators for good or for bad and permeate stories, points of view, decisions, and intentions, we turn to an exercise on emotions. If you are to listen to the feelings and emotions of clients, you first should be familiar with your own emotional states and your own style of emotional expression. This exercise is about your emotional style.

1. A lot has been written recently about "emotional intelligence." Find an article that summarizes current thinking about emotional intelligence and its place in people's lives. You will soon discover that, for many, the concept of emotional intelligence covers a lot more than emotions. It is an answer to the question: What does adult maturity look like? But let's start with feelings and emotions. Answer the following question about yourself as an "emotional" person.

What role do emotions play in your life?

_____

_____

How effectively do you control or manage negative emotions such as anger or hurt?

_____

_____

Which emotions are hardest for you to manage? What happens?

_____

_____

What role do positive emotions such as eagerness, joy, and contentment play in your life?

_____

_____

Comment on this statement: There is no such thing as a perfect emotional style.

_____

_____

_____

23

2. A number of emotional states are listed below. You are asked to describe what you feel when you feel these emotions. Describe what you feel as *concretely* as possible: How does your body react? What happens inside you? What do you feel like doing? Consider the following examples.

Example 1 — Accepted:
When I feel accepted,
· I feel warm inside.
· I feel safe.
· I feel free to be myself.
· I feel like sitting back and relaxing.
· I feel I can let my guard down.
· I feel like sharing myself.
· I feel some of my fears easing away.
· I feel at home.
· I feel at peace.
· I feel my loneliness melting away.

Example 2 — Scared:
When I feel scared,
· my mouth dries up.
· my bowels become loose.
· there are butterflies in my stomach.
· I feel like running away.
· I feel very uncomfortable.
· I feel the need to talk to someone.
· I turn in on myself.
· I'm unable to concentrate.
· I feel very vulnerable.
· I sometimes feel like crying.

1. Choose three of the emotions listed below or others not on the list. Try your hand at the emotions you have difficulty with. It's important to listen to yourself when you are experiencing emotions that are not easy for you to handle.
2. Picture to yourself situations in which you have experienced each of these three emotions.
3. Then, as in the example above, write down on a sheet of paper what you experienced.
4. What feelings are you most likely to avoid? Why?

1. accepted	12. disappointed	23. lonely
2. affectionate	13. free	24. loving
3. afraid	14. frustrated	25. rejected
4. angry	15. guilty	26. respected
5. anxious	16. hopeful	27. sad
6. attracted	17. hurt	28. satisfied
7. bored	18. inferior	29. shocked
8. competitive	19. interested	30. shy
9. confused	20. intimate	31. superior
10. defensive	21. jealous	32. suspicious
11. desperate	22. joyful	33. trusting

The reason for this exercise is to sensitize yourself to the wide variety of ways in which clients express and name their feelings and emotions. Diversity in emotional expression style is the norm.

Although the feelings and emotions of clients (not to mention your own) are extremely important, sometimes helpers concentrate too much, or rather too exclusively, on them. Feelings and emotions need to be understood, both by helpers and by clients, in the *context* of the experiences and behaviors that give rise to them. On the other hand, when clients hide their feelings, both from themselves and from others, then it is necessary to listen carefully to cues indicating the existence of suppressed, ignored, or unmanaged emotions.

LISTENING THOUGHTFULLY TO CLIENTS' STORIES

Listening thoughtfully means identifying the key elements of clients' stories —experiences, thoughts, behaviors, and feelings —and the relationships among them. Thoughtful listening is a function of empathy.

EXERCISE 3.8: LISTENING FOR CORE MESSAGES

Core messages are the main points of a client's story. The ingredients of core messages are key experiences, key thoughts, and key behaviors, together with the key feelings or emotions associated with them. In this exercise, you are asked to "listen to" and identify the key experiences and behaviors that give rise to the client's main feelings.

1. Listen very carefully to what the client is saying.
2. Identify the client's key experiences, what he or she says is happening or has happened to him or her.
3. Identify the client's key thoughts—what is going through his/her mind.
4. Identify the client's key behaviors, what he or she is doing, not doing, or failing to do.
5. Identify the key feelings and emotions associated with these experiences and behaviors.

Example: A 27-year-old African American man is talking to a minister about a visit with his mother the previous day. He says, "I just don't know what got into me! She kept nagging me the way she always does, asking me why I don't visit her more often. I kept asking myself where did all of this come from. I knew I should have tried to reason with her or just say nothing, but, as she went on, I got more and more angry. (He looks away from the counselor down toward the floor.) I finally began screaming at her. I told her to get off my case. (He puts his hands over his face.) I can't believe what I did. I called her a bitch. (Shaking his head.) I called her a bitch several times and then I left and slammed the door in her face."

Key experiences: Mother's nagging.
Key thoughts: What have I done to deserve this? I should keep my mouth shut.
Key behaviors: Losing his temper, yelling at her, calling her a name, slamming the door in her face.
Feelings/emotions generated: He now feels embarrassed, guilty, ashamed, distraught, disappointed with himself, remorseful. (Note carefully: This man is not at this moment *expressing* anger. Rather he is talking *about* his anger, the way he lets his temper get away from him.)

Now do the same with the following cases.

1. A 40-year-old Hispanic woman, married with no children, has had several sessions with a counselor. She went because she was bored and felt that all the color had gone out of her life. In a later session she says this: "These counseling sessions have really done me a great deal of good! I've worked hard in these sessions, and it's paid off. I enjoy my work more. I actually look forward to meeting new people. My husband and I are talking more seriously and decently to each other. At times he's even tender toward me

25

the way he used to be. Now that I've begun to take charge of myself more and more, there's just so much more freedom in my life!"

Client's key experiences:

_____

_____

_____

Client's key thoughts:

_____

_____

_____

Client's key behaviors:

_____

_____

_____

How does the client feel about these experiences, thoughts, and behaviors?

_____

_____

_____

2. A 20-year-old Asian American male college student who has volunteered to work with struggling high school students finds that he is learning more than he imagined he would. He tells his college advisor what it's like: "These kids deal with problems I have never had to face. Some days we'll start by working on some bit of homework but before we're done they're talking about being afraid of the gangs on the way to and from school. This one kid starts and ends each day by helping his mom who has MS. In the morning he gets her up and dresses her and in the evening he gets her ready for bed. Some days I do as much listening as talking. I go home wondering about my own life. I get embarrassed when I think of the ways I whine about my own problems. Many of these kids have a type of maturity about them you don't see in people who have lived as comfortably as I have. Boy do I have a lot to learn!"

Client's key experiences:

_____

_____

_____

Client's key thoughts:

_____

_____

_____

Client's key behaviors:

_____

_____

_____

How does the client feel about these experiences, thoughts, and behaviors?

_____

3. A 38-year-old woman, unmarried, talking about a situation with a friend: "My best friend has just turned her back on me. And I don't even know why! (said with great emphasis) From the way she acted, I think she has the idea that I've been talking behind her back. I simply have not! (also said with great emphasis) Damn! This neighborhood is full of spiteful gossips. She should know that. If she's been listening to those foul-mouthed jerks who just want to stir up trouble, she could at least tell me what's going on. I'm tempted to tell her to go jump in the lake. The nerve of her!"

Client's key experiences:

_____

_____

_____

Client's key thoughts:

_____

_____

Client's key behaviors:

_____

_____

How does the client feel about these experiences, thoughts, and behaviors?

_____

27

4. A 64-year-old Caucasian man, who has been told that he has terminal lung cancer, is speaking to a medical resident: "Why me? I'm not even that old! I keep looking for answers and there are none. I've sat for hours in church and I come away feeling empty. Why me? I don't smoke or anything like that. (He begins to cry.) Look at me. I thought I had some guts. I'm just a mess. Oh God, why terminal? What are these next months going to be like? (Pause, he stops crying.) Why would you care? I'm just a failure to you guys."

Client's key experiences:

_____

_____

_____

Client's key thoughts:

_____

_____

_____

Client's key behaviors:

_____

_____

_____

How does the client feel about these experiences, thoughts, and behaviors?

_____

THE SEARCH FOR MEANING

EXERCISE 3.9: PROCESSING WHAT YOU HEAR—THOUGHTFUL LISTENING

Listening in a thoughtful way goes beyond being able to recall what the client has said. It means being able to discriminate between the details of the client's story and the really meaningful points—the core messages. This exercise is done with a learning partner.

1. Read the section in the book entitled "Processing What You Hear: The Thoughtful Search for Meaning." Pay particular attention to the extended example of Denise and Jennie.
2. Take the role of the client and *through dialogue* discuss a problem or unused opportunity from your own life with a learning partner. Spend 10 to 15 minutes in the dialogue. Video the session.
3. When you have finished, each of you should jot down separately what you believe are the core messages. As you watch the video, compare what you have written. Ask yourself questions like these: How well did I capture my partner's core messages? How accurate was I? What messages did I miss? What caused me to miss any given message?
4. Reverse roles and repeat the exercise.

EXERCISE 3.10: LISTENING TO CLIENTS' COGNITIVE BEHAVIOR

A lot of things go on inside clients' heads. And so, although it is important to listen to their behavior, it is just as important to listen to this second set of behaviors inside. Clients make assumptions, develop points of view (including prejudices), make judgments, engage in the internal behavior leading to making decisions, formulate reasons to act, formulate explanations for actions they do take, and daydream, among other things. The stories they tell about themselves reveal a great deal about this internal behavior. Probing and empathy are skills that help you ferret out and understand this inner world. Listening to and understanding internal behavior helps us understand external behavior. Listen to the case and then answer the questions about the client's internal behavior.

Case 1. A husband and wife have entered counseling to help them deal more effectively with their daughter. The daughter is fifteen and is struggling in school and becoming involved with older boys. At this point the husband says: "It seems to me that we both need to stay on top of her school work. We need to do a better job of that—no question. But I think that at this stage the culture being spewed out by the media is raising her more than we are. I don't even know how much control we have anymore. This business about her relationships with boys, though, I think should be handled primarily by you, her mother. I'll back up whatever needs to be said but there is a part of this which is best handled between two women. For this one, I'll sit on the sidelines and come when needed. I don't trust boys her age. Not in this culture. She might react negatively to what you have to say, but I think she'd be even more negative with me."

Name some of the things that are going on inside the husband's head.

_____

_____

_____

_____

_____

What do you think is key?

_____

_____

_____

2. A single parent talks to a school counselor about the fact that his son is being picked on by others in his class. He has discussed the facts of the matter and feels the counselor has a good grasp of what is going on. Here is what he has to say: "If nothing is done, I'll have to take matters into my own hands and talk with the parents of the other boys. But that's not what I would prefer. This is a school matter and I will work with you and the teachers to see if this can be resolved in a sensible way. And don't tell me that 'boys will be boys,' because this has gone too far already. I hate seeing him coming home so miserable. I think back to when I was in school. We didn't have any of this nonsense. So what's going on? You people should be on top of all of this. I certainly cannot imagine my boy doing anything to provoke other boys. That's not his style."

29

Name some of the things that are going on inside the parent's head.

_____

_____

_____

_____

What do you think is key?

_____

_____

_____

3. A 33-year-old unmarried woman has recently learned that she is HIV-positive. "When I first learned about this I was devastated. The end. The curtain is coming down. But one morning I woke up and said to myself, 'Do something.' I did. I got on the net and learned everything I could about this. I spent days studying it. And, you know, I'm going to beat it. I'm going to get physically fit. I'm going to get my head together. I'm going to take the drugs that keep you going. I'm not sure how I'm going to afford them, but I'll get them. I'm going to volunteer for some experimental approaches. I don't know how you get on the list, but somehow I will. I'm going to beat this thing."

Name some of the things that are going on inside the woman's head.

_____

_____

_____

_____

_____

What do you think is key?

_____

_____

_____

LISTENING THOUGHTFULLY FOR OPPORTUNITIES

Spotting and understanding clients' opportunities is just as important as understanding their problems. Often exploiting opportunities is the best way to manage problems. Therefore, active listening includes listening for possible opportunities, which if pursued would help clients manage problem situations more effectively.

30

EXERCISE 3.11: LISTENING TO KEY OPPORTUNITIES

The instructions for this exercise are the same as those for the previous exercise.

Case 1. Ken, a 45-year-old African American man, has just been passed up for a promotion. He is talking with his supervisor who was a strong supporter. He starts by talking about his disappointment. But his supervisor points out that staying in his present position will allow him to see a project he started through to completion. Ken shifts his focus to the opportunity side of the event: "You may have a point. In fact, during my entire career I've been so focused on my next job that I've tended to do a lot of switching horses in mid-stream—taking new jobs before projects were really completed. Don't get me wrong. I'm not giving up on seeking promotions around here. But, I like what I'm doing and now I can give it my undivided energy. I suppose that people have to see that I can see things through, that I can get results with the best of them. Moving too quickly in the past has prevented them from seeing me at my best."

What is the opportunity?

_____

_____

What are the upside and the downside?

_____

_____

_____

How does Ken feel about it?

_____

_____

Case 2. A 43-year-old Caucasian woman has suffered a major financial setback in her small consulting business. She has just been offered a good position in a large consulting firm. "Lots of people would jump at this offer. The firm is solid, the job is challenging, and the pay is good. I'm really tempted. But I have really enjoyed being my own boss and building something out of nothing. If I take the offer, I'll have a boss again. Though I suppose that the economy has been my boss. The downturn is killing me. The little guys are the first to lose business. I do like the security I would have in the new job. But I know I won't be able to be as creative as I am when I'm on my own."

What is the opportunity?

_____

_____

What are the upside and the downside?

_____

_____

_____

31

How does she feel about it?

_____

_____

UNDERSTANDING CLIENTS' PROBLEMS AND OPPORTUNITIES THROUGH CONTEXT

EXERCISE 3.12: USING CONTEXT FOR THOUGHTFUL PROCESSING

Becoming a thoughtful processor requires two things — following the main points of the clients' stories (point of view, decision, or intention) as they unfold *and* at the same time placing it in the context of their lives. This exercise is designed to demonstrate the power of context.

1. Reread in the text "Processing What You Hear: The Thoughtful Search for Meaning."
2. Share a problem or unexploited opportunity from your own life with a learning partner. Provide no background or context during the conversation.
3. Discuss the issue for five to ten minutes.
4. When you have finished, tell your partner about the circumstances of your life that give added meaning to what you have shared. Discuss how the context changes the meaning of the problem or unexploited opportunity.
5. Reverse roles and give your learning partner a chance to do the same thing.

Example. A counseling trainee who is a veteran from the conflict in Afghanistan, 26, discusses how difficult it is to get back into the mainstream of society—family, community, culture, and now a professional education program. He talks about how a military mindset keeps stalking him. For instance, many of the things he is now doing seem trivial in comparison to battlefield demands. He says, "In some significant ways I'm still in Afghanistan." He finds that engaging in leisure activities, such as watching television or going to a movie with his girlfriend puts him on edge. He does not have the symptoms that go with PTSD—no "jitters, no nightmares," he says—but he just does not feel right.

Context. This counseling trainee comes from a Quaker background. He feels that some of his family members were disappointed when he joined the army and even more disappointed when he went to Afghanistan. But no one said anything to him. When he came home at the end of his first tour of duty, he was welcomed, certainly, but his community—family and friends—seemed different. Was *he* different or did *they* feel differently about him? He joined the army not because he was a great patriot, but because he thought he had to do something meaningful for others "on the big screen." He felt guilty about being "a person of privilege" and wanted to help people who were suffering in ways he never dreamed of. But he did not share these sentiments with anyone. Keeping things to yourself had been part of the culture of his community.

Discuss with a partner how this context colors his story. Then carry out the exercise.

THE SHADOW SIDE OF LISTENING

Since effective helpers are active listeners, it helps to learn about your own listening style — both the upside and the downside.

EXERCISE 3.13: FINDING THE SHADOW SIDE OF YOUR LISTENING STYLE

In this exercise you are asked to take an objective look at your style of listening and the way you process what you hear.

1. What kind of active listener are you? Give a brief, balanced description.

_____

_____

_____

_____

_____

_____

2. Re-read "The Shadow Side of Listening to Clients." Indicate below any areas of listening you think you should work on.

_____

_____

_____

_____

_____

3. Discuss your description of yourself as a listener and processor together with your shadow-side self-assessment with a learning partner. Talk about the implications of your shadow-side traits. Indicate possible actions you can take to overcome whatever deficiencies you discover.

Chapter 4

EMPATHIC RESPONDING: WORKING AT MUTUAL UNDERSTANDING

The payoff of attending and listening lies in the ability to communicate to clients an understanding of their stories, points of view, decisions, and intentions, together with the feelings and emotions they generate. Responding with empathy to the key messages the client is trying to get across is one way of communicating your understanding. It is one important way in which you translate the *value* of empathy discussed in Chapter 2 into behavior. Responding with empathy is a skill you need throughout the helping model. It is critical for establishing and developing relationships with clients, helping them clarify both problem situations and unexploited opportunities, setting goals, and developing and implementing strategies and plans. Read Chapter 4 in the text before doing the following exercises.

EXERCISE 4.1: CONFUSING SUBJECTIVE EMPATHY WITH INTERPERSONAL EMPATHY

What do people in general think of when they hear the term "empathy"? Read the vast literature on empathy and you will soon discover that there are many possible answers to that question. However, in *The Skilled Helper* empathy means *interpersonal empathy*, the ability to get inside a client's frame of reference and understand what the client is thinking and feeling together with the ability to communicate this understanding without prejudice to the client. Subjective empathy is different. As Clarke (2010a) notes, subjective empathy enables a person who is talking to another person to momentarily identify with that person through instinctive reactions and fleetingly imagine and experience what it is like to be a client" (p. 349). This kind of understanding of the client comes from the understanding of oneself and one's exposure in reality or in imagination to experiences similar to those of the client.

Let's say that you are with a client who is a victim of torture. The torture ended months ago, but the experience is still alive in him. In staying in touch with what is happening in the world, you have read accounts of horrific torture. You avoid reading such accounts now because the first hint of torture sends chills down your spine and gives rise to feelings of utter helplessness. As your client recounts his experiences, these feelings flood into you. But the client also talks about how his experience of torture has made him afraid to meet new people or even reconnect with old friends because he feels that the torture has scarred him psychologically and made him "ugly," even though physically he is not ugly at all.

1. What might your supervisor say if your first response to him was something like this? "When you began telling me what they did to you, I had to keep myself from shaking. I almost wanted you to stop."

_____

_____

2. Comment on the following response: "So the horror of all this is still so alive that reconnecting with your world seems practically impossible."

_____

_____

3. In what ways might subjective empathy help the therapy process?

_____

_____

4. In what ways might subjective empathy hinder the helping process?

_____

_____

5. Discuss in class or with a learning partner the distinctions among compassion, sympathy, and subjective empathy, especially as they relate to interpersonal empathy, and their possible roles in therapy.

EXERCISE 4.2: IDENTIFYING CORE MESSAGES IN CLIENTS' STORIES

The rest of these exercises deal with interpersonal empathy. In this exercise, you are asked to identify clients' key experiences, behaviors, and/or feelings and then translate them into a core message each client is trying to communicate.

1. Listen carefully to the client's statement.
2. Identify key experiences, behaviors, and the feelings they generate.
3. Pull them together in a statement of the client's core message.
4. After finishing, compare your responses with those of your learning partner. Then see if the two of you can improve upon your combined responses.

Example: Roula is recovering from a bad car accident in a rehabilitation facility. She is a week or two into a program that could well go on for a few months. In talking with one of the rehabilitation specialists, she says, "You told me it would be tough going. And I thought that I had prepared myself for it. I thought I had some courage in me. But now I can't find any grit at all. Doing even the smallest things takes so much effort! I keep breaking down and crying when I'm alone. I just keep giving in. . . . I'm just inches down a path that seems miles long. It seems endless."

Key experience(s): finding the rehabilitation program so difficult
Key behavior(s): failing to tap into the courage she thought she had; giving in to discouragement
Key feelings/emotions: disappointment, discouragement, despair

Core message: Roula seems disappointed almost to the point of despair because she has failed to tap into the "stuff" within her that would keep her going during a very tough rehabilitation program.

Now do the same for the following cases.

1. This woman is about to go to her daughter's graduation from college. She is talking with one of the ministers of her church: "I never thought that my daughter would make it through. I've invested a lot of money in her education. It meant scrimping and saving and not having some of the things I wanted. But money is certainly not the issue. More to the point, I've put a lot of emotion into making this day happen. I had to do a lot of hand-holding to help her get through. There were times when neither of us thought this day would come. But the day has arrived!"

35

Key experience(s):

_____

_____

Key behavior(s):

_____

_____

Key feelings/emotions:

_____

_____

Core message:

_____

_____

2. This older man has just had his wallet stolen. He became disoriented and was taken to a hospital. He's talking with a social worker. "I had just cashed my paycheck and the money was in the wallet. I've had a streak of bad luck. My sister was in an auto accident last week. And I was on my way to visit my nephew. Ironically, he was detained by the police for a minor theft earlier this week. Now he's probably thinking I've given up on him, when I haven't. There has not been much good news at all for a while."

Key experience(s):

_____

_____

Key behavior(s):

_____

_____

Key feelings/emotions:

_____

_____

Core message:

_____

_____

3. This woman is waiting for the results of medical tests. She is talking to a hospital volunteer: "I've been losing weight for about two months and feeling tired and listless all the time. I'm afraid of what these tests are going to say. I know I've been putting them off. I just hate hospitals and this kind of stuff. Well, now the waiting is getting to me. I . . . well, I just don't know where I stand. Nobody said anything to me during the tests. I don't think that's a good sign. It's all so impersonal, anyway."

Key experience(s):

_____

_____

Key behavior(s):

_____

_____

Key feelings/emotions:

_____

_____

Core message:

_____

_____

4. A client's prospective employer has just found out that the client has a criminal record: "I had hoped that I would get the job and prove myself before anyone found out about my record. I guess I was just stupid. I've just received a call from him telling me that I'm no longer being considered for the job. Well, I did what I thought was right. I never had the intention of deceiving anyone. I mean that I didn't think that I was doing anything wrong. . . . Well, even though I'm branded because of my record, I'm going to make it, somehow. I have to."

Key experience(s):

_____

_____

Key behavior(s):

_____

_____

Key feelings/emotions:

_____

_____

Core message:

_____

_____

5. This woman has just lost a custody case for her only son. During the interview with a counselor she seems almost in a daze: "I never dreamed that the court would award custody to my husband. I may not be a perfect mother, but I've done all the work in raising him so far. My husband has done nothing but give me a hard time over the years. He's so selfish and spiteful. I've been racking my brains trying to come up with something I can do. . . . Now he's won. . . . It's all over."

Key experience(s):

_____

_____

Key behavior(s):

_____

_____

Key feelings/emotions:

_____

_____

Core message:

_____

_____

EXERCISE 4.3: USING A "FORMULA" TO COMMUNICATE EMPATHY

Empathy focuses on the client's core messages—key experiences and/or key behaviors, key points of view, key decisions, key intentions—plus the feelings and emotions they generate. In this exercise you are asked to use the formula explained in the text: "You feel . . ." (followed by the right emotion and some indication of its intensity) "because . . ." (followed by the key experiences and/or behaviors that give rise to the emotion).

Please note that the use of a "formula" is merely a starting place to learn and practice the skill. It should not be taken literally; counseling cannot be reduced to formulas. In the next exercise (4.4), you will build on this skill by putting it in your own words.

1. Identify for yourself the speaker's key experiences, behaviors, points of view, decisions, intentions, and the feelings associated with them.
2. Formulate an empathic response. Even though you are writing the response, picture yourself actually talking to the person.

Example: A woman in a self-help group is talking about a relationship with a man. She says: "About a couple of months ago, he began being abusive, calling me names, describing my defects. To tell you the truth, that's why I joined this group, but I haven't had the courage to talk about it till now. The couple times I've tried to stand up for myself, he became even more abusive. He hasn't hit me or anything, but, anyway. So I've been just taking it, just sitting there taking it . . . like a dog or something. Do you think that this is just his bizarre way of getting rid of me? Why doesn't he just tell me?"

Key experience(s): being abused by companion, escalation in abuse
Key behavior(s): trying to stand up for herself, becoming passive, trying to figure out if this is his way of getting rid of her
Key feelings/emotions: distraught, confused, angry
Empathic response (using formula): You feel angry and confused because the abuse came from out of the blue and now you're wondering whether this is just his strange way of ending the relationship.

1. A first-year college student is talking to a counselor in the Center for Student Services. She has been talking about some of the difficulties of adjusting to college life. She comes from a small town and is attending a large state university. She speaks openly and seems to be in good spirits; she even smiles at times: "My new friends seem so much worldlier and confident than me. Most of them have traveled out of the country, have the latest greatest smartphones and computers, and act like college is no big deal. I mean, I am the first one in my family to go to college and sometimes I feel like I landed on the moon! This IS a big deal for me, plus I don't want to let my family down. I think with a little help I can figure it out, but right now I just feel like the only one who doesn't have it figured out yet – like I am playing catch-up."

38

Key experience(s):

_____

_____

Key behavior(s):

_____

_____

Key feelings/emotions:

_____

_____

Empathic response (formula)

_____

_____

2. A 66-year-old man is talking to a mental health counselor: "My wife died last year, and this year my youngest son went away to college. The other children are married. So now that I'm retired, I spend a lot of time rambling around a house that's . . . . (pauses, looks out the window for a while) . . . really too big for me. . . . You know, when I was working, there was a certain fullness to life. I always knew what to do. I, well . . . I made a difference. Now that I've got a comfortable retirement, I . . . ."

Key experience(s):

_____

_____

Key behavior(s)·

_____

_____

Key feelings/emotions:

_____

_____

Empathic response (formula):

_____

_____

3. This 33-year-old woman has been working with a counselor to find ways of handling sex discrimination at work. The company seems to preach one philosophy but implement another. Up to this point she has had some modest success, but now she wants to discuss a setback: "It seems they let me push as long as I stayed with the little stuff and did it quietly. But last week I brought up discrimination in our monthly team meeting . . . and my boss clammed up. And he's not one of the worst offenders. He's been quite cool since then and always seems to be busy. All of a sudden there's quite a different atmosphere in the office."

Key experience(s):

_____

_____

Key behavior(s):

_____

_____

Key feelings/emotions:

_____

_____

Empathic response (formula):

_____

_____

4. A young woman, 25, is talking about her current boyfriend with a counselor: "I can't quite figure him out. I still can't tell if he really cares about me, or if it's just about sex. It leaves everything up in the air. He's pleasant enough, but I'm not finding the substance that I thought was there. I do try to talk about serious things, things that interest me like what's happening in the world. The next thing I know we're back into trivia. I've been tempted to talk about this directly, but something holds me back."

Key experience(s):

_____

_____

Key behavior(s):

_____

_____

Key feelings/emotions:

_____

_____

Empathic response (formula):

_____

_____

5. This young man has just been abandoned by his wife after only a year of marriage: "We've been married for about a year. . . . She left a note saying that this has not been working out. Just like that. You know, I thought that things were going fairly well. Not perfect, of course. We had our ups and downs, but everyone does. Maybe I was so busy at work that there were things I didn't notice. I don't know if there's someone else. I really don't know why. . . . I must really sound stupid. I have no idea what to do to get her back. You can't make someone love you."

Key experience(s):

_____

_____

Key behavior(s):

_____

_____

Key feelings/emotions:

_____

_____

Empathic response (formula):

_____

_____

EXERCISE 4.4: USING YOUR OWN WORDS IN EMPATHIC RESPONSES

In this exercise you are asked to do two things:
1. First, use the "you feel . . . because . . ." formula to communicate understanding to the client.
2. Then recast your response in your own words while still identifying both the "feel" and the "because" part of empathy

Example: A married woman, 31, is having a "solo" meeting with a marriage counselor to review how things have been going from her point of view. At one point she says: "I can't believe it! You know when Tom and I were here last week we made a contract that said that he would be home for supper every evening and on time. Well, he came home on time every day this past week. I never dreamed that he would live up to his part of the bargain so completely! I've even begun making better meals!"

Formula. "You feel great because he really stuck to the contract!"
Non-formula. "Making good on his word has given you quite a boost!"

3. Now imagine yourself listening intently to each of the clients quoted below. First use the "You feel . . . because . . ." formula; then use your own words. Try to make the second response sound as natural (as much like yourself) as possible. After you use your own words, check to see if you have both a "you feel" part and a "because" part in your response.

1. A 28-year-old woman is talking about her job with a colleague: "It's not a big thing. But this is the third time this month I've been asked to change hours with her. I said yes, of course. But it certainly seems to indicate who is more important there. Why does it always have to be me who defers to her?"

Use the formula.

_____

_____

41

Use your own words.

_____

_____

2. A man who has been suffering from depression for a number of months is talking with a psychologist: "I've seen my doctor a couple of times. But now, since the depression isn't getting any better, he wants to give me this drug. . . . But I don't even take aspirin if I don't have to. Somehow drugs and I don't mix. If I had pneumonia or some infection, it would be one thing. But this is all in my head. I don't want to be taking psycho medication. I'm not crazy!"

Use the formula.

_____

_____

Use your own words.

_____

_____

3. A counseling trainee is talking to her instructor. The training group has just been introduced to the skill of inviting clients to challenge themselves. They have practiced self-challenge and have just begun using invitations to self-challenge with one another: "For the first time in this program I am having trouble and it's bothering me. What I've found out is that I have no problem with self-challenge. In some ways I have been doing that for years. But now I see that maybe I've been picking on myself, you know, being too much of a perfectionist. And I'm finding it really hard to challenge the members of my group. Oh, I know the theory. But doing it is hard. It's almost as if they won't like me if I do it well."

Use the formula.

_____

_____

Use your own words.

_____

_____

4. A fellow trainee has been talking with you about the counselor training program. He calls you up and says he wants to talk with you right away. When you meet, he says: "You know, tomorrow we're going to start talking about our own problems. Well, the kinds of things that could stand in the way of being good helpers. . . . Well, there are things I'd rather not say in the group. . . . I barely had the courage to talk with you. . . . You know, a couple of issues I'd rather not talk about _could_ stand in the way of my being the kind of counselor I should be. . . . But I'm just not ready. I could be dishonest."

Use the formula.

_____

_____

Use your own words.

_____

_____

5. A man, Frank, is being forced out of the company where he has held a senior position for almost twenty years: "It came out of nowhere. I came in two days ago and there on my desk was a notice from the venture capital group that bought us saying that I was terminated. It was as impersonal as that. . . . I kept reading it over and over again like I was in some dream. I tried to call my boss but couldn't get her. Later I found out that she had been let go, too. The notice said I get some outplacement help. What kind of word is that! It's a fancy word for dumping."

Use the formula.

_____

_____

Use your own words.

_____

_____

EXERCISE 4.5: EMPATHIC RESPONSES WITH CLIENTS FACING DILEMMAS

Clients often talk about complicated issues. When this is the case, it is essential to listen even more carefully in order to pick up and respond to core messages. For example, clients often talk about conflicting values, complicated experiences, behaviors, points of view, decisions, intentions, and complex emotions. Responding with empathy means picking up the uncertainties and communicating an understanding of the conflict.

1. Identify the conflict or dilemma.
2. Use the empathic response formula to communicate understanding.
3. Express the response in your own words.

Example: A 32-year-old woman is talking to a counselor about adopting a child: "I'm going back and forth, back and forth. I say to myself, 'I really want a child,' but then I think about Bill [her husband] and his reluctance. He really wants our own child and is so reluctant to raise someone else's. We don't even know why we can't have children. But the fertility specialists don't offer us much hope. At times when I really want to be a mother I think I should marry someone who would be willing to adopt a child. But I love Bill and don't want to point an accusing finger at him."

The conflict or dilemma. She believes that she runs the risk of alienating her husband if she insists on adopting a child, even though she strongly favors adoption.
Formula. "You feel trapped between your desire to be a mother and your love for your husband."
You own words. "You're caught in the middle. Adopting a child would solve your problem but perhaps create one for your husband."

1. A 30-year-old factory worker is talking to a counselor about his job: "Work is okay. I do make a good living, and both my family and I like the money. Me and my wife are both from poor homes, and we're

43

living much better than we did when we were growing up. But the work I do is the same thing day after day. I may not be the world's brightest person, but there's a lot more to me than just running those machines."

The conflict.

_____

_____

Empathic response (formula):

_____

_____

Your own words.

_____

_____

2. A mental hospital patient, 54, who has spent five years in the hospital, is talking to the members of an ongoing therapy group. Some of the members have been asking him what he's doing to get out. He says, "I don't know why you're trying to push me out of here. To tell the truth, I like it here. I'm safe and secure. So why are so many people here so damn eager to see me leave? . . . Is it a crime because I feel comfortable here? (Pause, then in a more conciliatory voice.) I know you're all interested in me. I see that you care. But do I have to please you by doing something I don't want to do?"

The conflict.

_____

_____

The formula.

_____

_____

Your own words.

_____

_____

3. A juvenile probation officer is speaking to a colleague: "These kids drive me up the wall. Sometimes I think I'm really stupid for doing this kind of work. They taunt me. They push me as far as they can. To some of them I'm just another 'pig.' But every time I think of quitting—and this gets me—I know I'd miss the work and even miss the kids one way or another. When I wake up in the morning, I know the day's going to be full and it's going to demand everything I've got."

The conflict.

_____

_____

The formula.

_____

_____

Your own words.

_____

_____

EXERCISE 4.6: SEEING YOURSELF ON VIDEO

One of the benefits of the universal availability of video is that you can see yourself in action. Extensive use of video is a must in training programs. Because empathy is such an important therapeutic communication skill, seeing how well you respond with empathy is a good place to start.

1. View a video of someone who is a master at communicating empathy. On YouTube you will find a video of Carl Rogers in a therapy session with Gloria, the client. He makes extensive use of empathy in this session.
2. Prepare for the video session by choosing some problem situation with which you are currently grappling, one that you are willing to speak about with a learning partner. Your partner will do the same.
3. Before turning on the video, the client should say a few words to put his or her problem situation in context.
4. Roll the camera and engage in a 10-15 minute session in which you respond to the client almost exclusively with empathy, as Rogers does in the Gloria video.
5. After the session, take the lead in giving yourself feedback as you and your learning partner debrief the session. What have you learned from watching yourself?
6. Reverse roles and repeat the entire process.

EXERCISE 4.7: RESPONDING WITH EMPATHY IN EVERYDAY LIFE

If communicating empathy is to become a part of your natural communication style, you will have to practice it outside formal training sessions. That is, it must become part of your everyday communication style or it will tend to lack genuineness in helping situations. Practicing empathic communication "out there" is a relatively simple process.

1. **The improbability of empathic responding.** Responding to others with empathy is not a normative response in everyday conversations, even among people who otherwise put into practice the value of empathy. For instance, sometimes people use phrases such as "I know how you are feeling" or "I get you" or minimal encouragers like "oh-uh-huh" to convey empathy, but these phrases may not truly express empathy. Find this out for yourself. Observe everyday conversations. Count how many times interpersonal empathy is used as a response in any given conversation.
2. **Your own use of empathy.** Next try to observe how often you yourself use empathy as part of your normal style. In the beginning, don't necessarily try to increase the number of times you do so. Merely observe your usual behavior. What part does empathic responding normally play in your interpersonal communication style?
3. **Increasing your empathic responses.** Begin to increase the number of times you respond to others with empathy. Be as natural as possible. Do not overwhelm others with this response; rather try to incorporate it gradually into your style. You will probably discover that there are quite a few opportunities for responding with empathy without being phony. Find some way of keeping track of your progress.

45

4. **The impact of empathy.** Observe the impact your use of empathy has on others. Don't use others for the purpose of experimentation, but, as you gradually increase your use of this communication skill naturally, notice how it influences and enriches your conversations. What impact does it have on you? What impact does it have on others?

5. **Learnings.** In a forum set up by the instructor, discuss with your fellow trainees what you are learning from this experiment.

If responding with empathy becomes part of your communication style "out there," then you should appear more and more natural in doing so in the training program, both in playing the role of the helper and in listening and providing feedback to your fellow trainees. On the other hand, if you use empathy only in the training sessions, it will most likely remain artificial.

Chapter 5

THE ART OF PROBING AND SUMMARIZING

Problems and opportunities are better managed when they are clear and specific. If Connie and Chuck want to deal with the poor communication they have with each other in their marriage, then the key issues relating to communication need to be spelled out in terms of specific experiences, behaviors, points of view, decisions, intentions, and feelings in specific situations. Clients need to focus on concrete rather than abstract issues. Counselors use probes to help clients "fill in the picture," turning vague statements into concrete and specific ones. Vaguely described problems lead only to vague solutions. Read Chapter 5 in *The Skilled Helper* before doing these exercises. This section has three parts: problem and opportunity clarity, probing, and summarizing.

PROBLEM AND OPPORTUNITY CLARITY

EXERCISE 5.1: SPEAKING CONCRETELY ABOUT PROBLEMS AND UNUSED OPPORTUNITIES

This exercise is designed to help you get a feel for both vagueness and concreteness. In this exercise you are asked to focus on your own story in terms of your own experiences, behaviors, points of view, decisions, intentions, and feelings.

1. Give one vague statement of some problem situation.
2. Give one vague statement of some unused opportunity.
3. Turn each vague statement into a concrete and specific statement in terms of key experiences, behaviors, points of view, decisions, intentions, and feelings.
4. Focus on issues that can make a difference in your life.

Example 1: Problems: Karen writes about her need to control situations.

Vague statement of problem situation: "I tend to be a bit domineering at times."
Concrete statement: "I try, usually in subtle ways, to get others to do what I want to do. I even pride myself on this. In conversations, I take the lead. I interrupt others, jokingly and in a good-natured way, but I make my points. If a friend is talking about something serious when I'm not in the mood to hear it, I change the subject."

Example 2: Unused Opportunity: Austin, in his fourth year of a doctoral program in clinical psychology, has also taken a couple of courses in organizational psychology. He has just finished his internship.

Vague statement of possible opportunity: "One thing I learned during my internship rotations is that mental-health organizations are not what they could be. But I'm not sure I can do anything about it without violating my commitment to people."
Concrete statement: "The organizational psychology courses I took made it clear to me that some mental-health centers are poorly-run organizations. Even with a little background I knew some things I could do to help them be more efficient and effective. In fact, the whole area of applying effective management and organizational ideas to mental-health systems appeals to me enormously. But I feel guilty about pursuing that possibility after graduation. It's like betraying the reasons for going into clinical psych in the first place — mainly to help others. I really liked dealing with individuals and groups during my internship, but I was distracted by how poorly these places are run. A number of clinical psychologists I met thought that administration was for the birds, you know, for lesser people."

47

In the spaces below, explore two issues that are related to some problem situation or situations of your own. Try to choose issues that might affect the quality of your helping.

1. Vague statement: Problem

_____

_____

Concrete statement.

_____

_____

_____

_____

_____

_____

2. Vague statement: Unused Opportunity.

_____

_____

Concrete statement.

_____

_____

_____

_____

_____

_____

Share these with a learning partner. Get feedback on how clear your second statement is. If you do not think that your partner's statement is as clear as it might be, use probes to help him or her make the statement clearer.

PROBES

EXERCISE 5.2: PROBING FOR KEY ISSUES AND CLARITY

A probe is a statement or a question that invites a client to discuss an issue more fully. In Exercise 5.1 you were asked to probe yourself. Probes are ways of getting at important details that clients do not think of or are reluctant to talk about. They can be used at any point in the helping process to clarify and explore

48

issues, search for missing data, expand perspectives, and point toward possible client actions. Of course, an overuse of probes can lead to gathering a great deal of irrelevant information. The purpose of a probe is not data for its own sake, but information—experiences, behaviors, points of view, decisions, intentions, and feelings—that serve the process of problem management and opportunity development.

In this exercise, you will be presented brief problem situations with a bit of context. Your job is to formulate possible probes to help clients move forward in the helping process.

1. First, use empathic responses to understand the client.
2. Next, formulate a probe that might help the client further identify or explore key issues, experiences, behaviors, points of view, decisions, intentions, and feelings.
3. Briefly state how your probe might help the client move forward.

Example: A Caucasian man, 24, complains that he is severely tempted to go on experimenting sexually with women other than his wife: "Although I have not had an extended affair, I have had a few sexual encounters and feel that some day I might have an affair. I don't blame myself or my wife, though I'm not sure I'll ever find the kind of sexual satisfaction I want with her. I've never had such strong sexual urges. I thought that once I was married, the sexual thing would be taken care of. That's certainly not the way things have turned out. I'm not sure where I'm headed."

Empathic statement: "It sounds like your sexual urges are so strong right now that they're in the driver's seat. But you're puzzled and are not quite sure what all this means and where it's going."
Possible probe: "As to where it's going, what are some of the possibilities?"
How might it help the client move forward? To help the client begin thinking through some of the implications of the decisions he's made about his sexual life.

1. Grace, 19, an unmarried, first-year Caucasian college student, comes to counseling because of an unexpected and unwanted pregnancy: "Right now I realize that the father could be either of two guys. That probably says something about me right there. I'm not sure what I want to do about the baby. I haven't told my parents yet, but I think that they will be very upset, but in the end sympathetic. At least I hope so. But I've gotten myself into this mess and I have to get myself out."

Empathic statement.

_____

_____

Possible probe.

_____

_____

How might it help the client move forward?

_____

_____

2. You are a counselor in a halfway house. You are dealing with Tom, 44, who has just been released from prison where he served two years for armed robbery. This was his first encounter with the law. He has been living at the halfway house for two weeks. The halfway house experience is designed to help him reintegrate himself into society. Living in the house is voluntary. The immediate problem is that Tom

49

came in drunk a couple of nights ago. He was supposed to be out on a job-search day. Drinking is against the rules of the house. When you talk to him, he says "I know this looks bad. But I don't think it's as bad as it looks. There was no liquor inside prison. This was my first encounter with alcohol since I got out. I guess I just went overboard. I shouldn't have done it, but it's not the end of the world. Or it shouldn't be."

Empathic statement.

_____

_____

Possible probe.

_____

_____

How might it help the client move forward?

_____

_____

3. Arnie is a born-again Christian. He has begun to do a fair amount of informal preaching at his place of employment. While some of his co-workers sympathize with his views, others are turned off. Since he feels that he is being driven by a "clear vision," he becomes more and more militant. His supervisor has cautioned him a few times, but this has done little to change Arnie's behavior. Finally, he is given an ultimatum to talk to one of the counselors in the Employee Assistance Program about these issues or be suspended from his job. He says to the counselor, "I have a duty to spread the word. And if I have a duty to do so, then I also have the right. I'm a good worker. In fact, I believe in hard work. So it's not like I'm taking time off for the Lord's work. Now what's wrong with that?"

Empathic statement.

_____

_____

Possible probe.

_____

_____

How might it help the client move forward?

_____

_____

4. A trainee in the counselor training program makes this statement in his small group: "I do not take criticism well. When I receive almost any kind of negative feedback, I usually smile and seem to shrug it off, but inside I begin to pout. Also, deep inside, I put the person who gave me the feedback on a 'list.' Those on the list have to pay for what they did. I find this hard to admit, even to myself. It sounds so petty. For instance, two weeks ago in the training group I received some negative feedback from Cindy. I

felt angry and hurt because I thought she was my friend. Since then I've tried to see what mistakes she makes here. I've even felt a bit disappointed because I haven't been able to catch her in any kind of glaring mistake. It goes without saying that I'm embarrassed to say all this."

Empathic statement.

_____

_____

Possible probe.

_____

_____

How might it help the client move forward?

_____

_____

5. Renata is talking with a counselor about her relationship with her mother: "I feel guilty and depressed whenever my mother calls and implies that she's lonely. I then get angry with myself for giving in to guilt so easily. Then the whole day has a cloud over it. I get nervous and irritable and take it out on others. Or I brood. Sometimes it even interferes with my work. Then I do what I have to."

Empathic statement.

_____

_____

Possible probe.

_____

_____

How might it help the client move forward?

_____

_____

EXERCISE 5.3: EMPATHIC RESPONSES AND TWO KINDS OF PROBES

This exercise asks you to combine several skills—the ability to share understanding through empathic responses, to identify areas needing clarification, and to use both question-type and statement-type probes to help clients clarify their stories, points of view, decisions, and intentions, together with how they feel about all of these.

1. First, reply to the client with empathy.
2. Use a question-type probe in open-ended question form to help the client explore or clarify some issue.

3. Convert the question-type probe into a statement-type probe.
4. Indicate how the probe might help the client move forward.

Example: A 25-year-old law student is talking to a school counselor: "I learned yesterday that I've flunked out of school and that there's no recourse. I've seen everybody, but the door is shut tight. What a mess! I know I haven't gotten down to business the way I should. This is my first year in a large city and there are so many distractions. And school is so competitive. I have no idea how I'll face my parents. They've paid for my college education and this year of law school. I'll have to tell them that it's all down the drain."

Empathic response: "In your eyes the punishment doesn't seem to fit the crime. And it all sounds, not just desperate, but so final."
Question probe: "Which administrators did you see and which doors were shut?"
Statement probe: "I'm not sure who you mean by 'everybody' and it's not clear which doors are completely shut."
How might the probe help the client move forward? It might help the client identify possibilities that he has overlooked because of the emotionality surrounding the situation.

1. A high school senior to a school counselor: "My dad told me the other night that I looked relaxed. Well, that's a joke. I don't feel relaxed. There's a lull right now, because of semester break, but next semester I'm signed up for two math courses, and math really rips me up. But I need it for science since I want to go into pre-med."

Empathic response.

_____

_____

Question probe.

_____

_____

Statement probe.

_____

_____

How might it help the client move forward?

_____

_____

2. A 27-year-old Japanese American woman talking to a counselor about a relationship that has just ended (she speaks in a rather matter-of-fact voice): "About three weeks ago I came back from visiting my parents who live in Nevada and found a letter from my friend Gary. He said that he still loves me but that I'm just not the person for him. In the letter he thanked me for all the good times we had together these last three years. He asked me not to try to contact him because this would only make it more difficult for both of us. End of story. I guess I've let my world collapse. People at work have begun complaining about me. And I've been like a zombie most of the time."

52

Empathic response.

_____

_____

Question probe.

_____

_____

Statement probe.

_____

_____

How might it help the client move forward?

_____

_____

3. A married Latino man, 25 years old, is talking to a counselor about trouble with his mother-in-law: "The way I see it, she is really trying to destroy our marriage. She's so conniving. And she's very clever. It's hard to catch her in what she's doing. You know, it's rather subtle. Well, I've had it! If she's trying to destroy our marriage, she's getting pretty close to achieving her goal."

Empathic response.

_____

_____

Question probe.

_____

_____

Statement probe.

_____

_____

How might it help the client move forward?

_____

_____

4. A Caucasian man, 45 years old, who has just lost his wife and home in a tornado, has been talking about his loss to a social worker: "This happened to a friend of mine in Kansas about ten years ago. He never recovered from it. His life just disintegrated and nobody could do anything about it. . . . It was like the end of the world for him. You never think it's going to happen to you."

Empathic response.

_____

_____

Question probe.

_____

_____

Statement probe.

_____

_____

How might it help the client move forward?

_____

_____

EXERCISE 5.4: PROBING FOR ACTION

Remember that each interaction in the helping process should be, all things considered, some kind of stimulus for client action—the "little" actions, as it were—that precede formal action based on a plan. In this exercise you are asked to use both empathic responses and probes to help clients consider actions they might take to move forward. Probes are very useful in helping clients develop a solution-focused approach in the helping process.

Example. A 44-year-old divorced woman is talking to a counselor about her drinking. This is the second session. She has spent a lot of time telling her story. She has already admitted that she engages in evasions and sometimes simply lies about her problems. She says, "Actually, it's a relief to tell someone the truth. I don't have to give you any excuses or make the story sound right. I drink because I like to drink; I'm just crazy about the stuff, that's all. But I'm under no delusions that telling you is going to solve anything. When I get out of here, I know I'm going straight to a bar to drink. Some new bar, new faces, some place they don't know me."

Empathic response. "So, for you, drinking is a way of life. No use making excuses. That's the way it is. So you're headed to a bar."

Probe for action. "If a friend had heard you talking and challenged you by saying, 'Hey! You're better than this. Don't go to a bar. Do something constructive, something creative for a change,'" what could you do instead of going to the bar? What might one step in a different direction look like?"

1. A German American man, 57 years old, is talking to a counselor about a family problem: "My younger brother, he's 53, has always been a kind of bum. He's always poaching off the rest of the family. Last week my unmarried sister told me that she'd given him some money for a 'business deal.' Business deal, my foot! I'd like to get hold of him and give him a good kick! Oh, he's not a vicious guy. Just weak. He's never been able to get a fix on life. But he's got the whole family in turmoil now, and we can't keep going through hell because of him."

Empathic response.

_____

_____

Probe for action.

_____

_____

2. A 25-year-old graduate student is speaking to an instructor whom he trusts: "I have two term papers due tomorrow. I'm giving a report in class this afternoon. My wife is down with the flu. And now I find out that the program director wants to talk with me about my progress in the program. I've been working a couple of part-time jobs—I've got to just to keep things going. I know I'm behind, but I still think I can handle things. I hope they're not going to give me any kind of ultimatum."

Empathic response.

_____

_____

Probe for action.

_____

_____

3. An African American man, 49 years old, is talking to a rehabilitation counselor after an operation that has left him with one lung: "I'll never be as active as I used to be. But at least I'm beginning to see that life is still worth living. I have to take a long look at the possibilities, no matter how much they've narrowed. I can't explain it, but there's something good stirring in me. I'm not sure I'm making any sense to you."

Empathic response.

_____

_____

Probe for action.

_____

_____

4. Mark and Lisa, a married Caucasian couple, both 33 years old, have spent years attempting to have children and finally adopted a baby girl, Andrea. Their relationship, which until then seemed quite good, has begun to disintegrate. Mark has made some cracks about "the stranger in the house." Andrea has proved to be a somewhat difficult baby. Lisa feels exhausted and blames Mark for not helping her. They

55

are both thinking about divorce now, but feel very guilty because of the child. Both of them say, "If only we had never adopted Andrea."

Empathic response.

_____

_____

Probe for action.

_____

_____

EXERCISE 5.5: USING PROBES TO HELP OTHERS COMMUNICATE BETTER

This is an exercise that can be done both in the training group and in your everyday life. You most likely run into people who are not very good at dialogue. You can use probes to help them do better.

1. Find a person who is not a good communicator, someone not good at dialogue.
2. Use both empathic responses and probes to help this person engage in dialogue, that is, engage in turn taking, connecting with what you have to say, staying open to mutual influence, and, in the end, co-creating some kind of conversational outcome with you.
3. After you have engaged in a couple of these conversations, discuss your successes and your failures with a learning partner. What do you have to do to become better at helping people less gifted in communication engage in dialogue? Ultimately, this means using empathy and probes to help clients engage in dialogue as they tell their stories, reveal their points of view, discuss their decisions, and reveal their intentions.

Example. Trudy, a counselor trainee, is talking with Nathan, a friend of hers in the neighborhood. Nathan, who always has very strong opinions, has been talking almost nonstop about why he thinks that the government is going to make a big mistake by over-regulating the financial industry because of the financial debacle. Trudy uses the skills she is learning to try to help Nathan have a dialogue with her.

Nathan (continuing at a fast pace): Take compensation. Passing laws about how much people should be paid is not the function of government. Why not . . ..

Trudy (interrupting): Nathan, your main point seems to be government intervention just doesn't work. The times they've tried to run the banks, they've done a poor job. So that's what they shouldn't do. What do you think that government agencies should do? What would you do to make the financial industry more responsible?

Nathan: I'm not sure that I'd do anything. I mean I wish that the system would just straighten itself out. There are a lot of very smart people in finance.

Trudy: I don't doubt that, but if they are so smart, why did they let things get out of hand? A lot of the bankers have been admitting that mistakes have happened, even though they never seem to take personal responsibility for any of them.

Nathan: OK, mistakes—a lot of mistakes—were made, but why should big government make things worse by adding their own mistakes? We'd lose our financial leadership position. Let me tell you how it works. . .

Trudy (interrupting): Who says that we have to be financial leaders? What about ethics? What about the common good? What about responsibility? I'm not sure what you mean by leadership.

56

Nathan: Leadership means the best. The most powerful. The most influential.

Trudy: It seems that the financial industry "influenced" a lot of people to get mortgages they could not afford.

Nathan: All right. I'm not trying to say that the financial industry is perfect. There are a lot of warts. What we need is some kind of balanced approach to reform. And I don't see that happening right now. Government is overwhelming the industry with new rules and regulations of dubious value.

Trudy: So "balance" is the important operating term. The question is, "How do we get the balance right?" It seems that a lot of different voices have to contribute to the solution.

Nathan: Yes, but we need to balance the power of the voices. We need focus. Don't get me wrong. I think that the common good should play an important role here, but we need to define what we mean by the common good.

Trudy: Yes, it sounds like we need to discuss a lot of things we take for granted. The common good is just one of them. Justice, fairness, equity, community—there's a lot of things we need to define if we are going to negotiate sensibly.

Nathan: There's a good word. Negotiate. Some of the ads about negotiation-skills programs seem to define negotiating as winning. That's not right.

Trudy: Yes, if it means winning, then you need to do whatever it takes to win. That's one of the things that got us into this mess in the first place.

Nathan: It seems that we need to take the whole financial system apart conceptually and then put it back together again. Lack of transparency and mutual understanding has caused a lot of trouble.

And on they go. Discuss Trudy's approach here with your learning partner. What did she do right? What did she do wrong? What could she have done to improve the quality of the dialogue?

SUMMARIZING

At a number of points throughout the helping process it is useful for helpers to summarize or to have clients summarize the principal points of their interactions. This places clients under pressure to focus and move on. Since summarizing can place pressure on clients to move forward, it is an invitation to self-challenge.

EXERCISE 5.6: SUMMARIZING AS A WAY OF PROVIDING FOCUS

This exercise assumes that trainees have been using the skills of sharing empathic responses and probing in order to help one another tell their stories, share their points of view, discuss their decisions, and spell out their intentions.

1. The total training group is divided into subgroups of three.
2. There are three roles in each subgroup: helper, client, and observer.
3. The helper spends about eight minutes counseling the client. The client should continue to explore one of the problem areas he or she has chosen to deal with in the training group.
4. At the end of four minutes, the helper summarizes the principal points of the interaction. Helpers should try to make the summary both accurate and concise. The helper can draw on past interactions if he or she is counseling a fellow trainee whom he or she has counseled before. At the end of eight minutes or so, the helper should engage in a second summary.
5. At the end of each summary, the helper should ask the client to draw some sort of implication or conclusion from the summary that helps the client move forward.

6. Then both observer and client give the helper feedback as to the accuracy and the helpfulness of the summaries provided. The summaries are useful if they help move the client toward problem clarification, goal setting, and action.

7. This process is repeated until each person in the subgroup has had an opportunity to play each role.

Example 1: It would be too cumbersome to print eight minutes of dialogue here, but consider this brief outline of a case. A young man, 22 years old, has been talking about some developmental issues. One of his concerns is that he sees himself as relating to women poorly. One side of his face is scarred from a fire that occurred two years previous to the counseling session. He has made some previous remarks about the difficulties he has relating to women. After four minutes of interaction, the helper summarizes:

HELPER: Dave, let me see if I have the main points you've been making. First, because of the scars, you think you turn women off even before you get to talk with them. The second point, and I have to make sure that this is what you are saying, is that your initial approach to women is cautious, or a bit cynical, or maybe even subtly hostile since you've come to expect rejection somewhat automatically.

DAVE: Yeah, but now that you've put it all together, I am not so sure that the hostility is all that subtle.

HELPER: So at least at times there is some open hostility. . . .You also said that the women you meet are cautious with you. Some might see you as a bit "nasty," I believe that was your word. Others steer clear of you because they see you as difficult to talk to and get to know. Finally, what closes the circle is that you interpret their caution as being turned off by your physical appearance.

DAVE: I don't like to hear it that way, but that's what I've been saying.

HELPER: If these points are fairly accurate, I wonder what implication you might see in them.

DAVE: Well, one possibility is that *I'm* the one that rejects me because of my face. If that's the case, then nothing's going to get better until I come to grips with myself.

Note that the client draws an implication from the summary ("I am the primary one who rejects me") and moves on to some minimal declaration of intent ("I need to change this").

Example 2: Artemis, a 37-year-old woman, has been talking about her lack of assertive behavior in a paraprofessional helper training group. She sees clearly that this lack of assertion stands in the way of being an effective helper. She and her helper explore this theme for a few minutes and then the helper invites her to give a summary of the main points she is making:

HELPER: "Artemis, it might help if you would pull together the main points you've been making. It might help us to see the way forward."

ARTEMIS: "Okay, let's see if I can pull this together. I'm convinced that the ability to move into the life of the client without apologizing for my assertiveness is essential. However, this simply has not been part of my normal interpersonal style. I don't intrude into the lives of others. If anything, I'm too hesitant to place demands on anyone. When I take the role of helper in training sessions, I feel awkward even sharing basic empathic responses and even more awkward using probes. As a result, I let my clients ramble and their problems remain unfocused. In social settings I'm quite passive, except now I'm much more aware of it.

HELPER: What implication might you draw from it?

TRAINEE: When I put it all together like that, my immediate reaction is to say that I shouldn't try to be a counselor. But I think I would be selling myself short. No matter what career I choose to follow, I need to become more assertive. I have to learn how to take risks with people.

The feedback from the client and the observer should center on the accuracy and the usefulness of the summary, not on a further exploration of the client's problem. Recall that feedback is most effective when it is clear, concise, behavioral, and nonpunitive.

Chapter 6

FACILITATING CLIENT SELF-CHALLENGE: FROM NEW PERSPECTIVES TO NEW BEHAVIOR

Chapter 6 in *The Skilled Helper* discusses the role of challenging in the helping process. Helping clients challenge themselves both to participate actively in the helping process and to act on what they learn adds great value. However, while challenge without understanding is abrasive, understanding without challenge is anemic. Before doing the following exercise, read Chapter 6.

We begin with an exercise in self-exploration focused on some normative developmental tasks. Many of the clients you see will be struggling with developmental concerns that all of us have struggled with or are currently working on. Like all of us, clients will have both strengths and "soft spots" in coping with the developmental tasks of life. Self-responsibility leading to self-challenge plays an important role in managing developmental tasks across the life span.

EXERCISE 6.1: A REVIEW OF SOME BASIC DEVELOPMENTAL TASKS

In this exercise, you are asked to consider your experience with ten major developmental tasks of life and do some soul searching. Developmental tasks that are not addressed effectively earlier in life have a way of hanging around and haunting us later.

1. Read through the list and then choose three areas where some self-challenge might be called for. Try to choose areas you think will have an impact on your career as counselor.

A. COMPETENCE. What do I do well? To what extent do I see myself as a person who is capable of getting things done? How effective am I in gathering the resources needed to accomplish the goals I set for myself? In what areas of life do I excel? In what areas of life would I want to be more competent than I am?

My Strengths
_____
_____
_____

My Soft Spots
_____
_____
_____

B. AUTONOMY: How well do I make it on my own? How effectively do I avoid being either overly dependent or too independent? To what degree am I reasonably interdependent in my work and social life? When I need help, how easy do I find it to ask for it? In what social settings do I find myself most dependent? counterdependent? independent? interdependent?

My Strengths

_____

_____

_____

My Soft Spots

_____

_____

_____

C. VALUES: What do I believe in and prize? What are my principal values? To what degree do I pursue reasonable development in my value system? How well do I put my values into practice? What value conflicts do I face? In what social settings do I pursue the values that are most important to me?

My Strengths

_____

_____

_____

My Soft Spots

_____

_____

_____

D. IDENTITY: Who am I in this world? To what extent do I have a sense of who I am and the direction I'm going in life? What kind of congruence exists between the way I see myself and the way others see me? What kind of "center" gives meaning to my life? In what social settings do I have my best feelings for who I am? In what social settings do I tend to lose a sense of who I am? In what ways am I confused or dissatisfied with who I am?

My Strengths

_____

_____

_____

My Soft Spots

_____

_____

_____

E. INTIMACY. What are my closer relationships like? What kinds of closeness do I have with others? To what extent are there degrees of closeness in my life — from acquaintances to friends to romantic relationships? What is intimacy in my peer group like? How well do I get along with others? What concerns do I have about my interpersonal life?

My Strengths

_____

_____

_____

My Soft Spots

_____

_____

_____

F. SEXUALITY. Who am I as a romantic/sexual person? If not currently in a romantic relationship, to what degree do I want a deep, stable, romantic relationship? In what ways do I look forward to some deeper stable relationship? What misgivings do I have about such a relationship? To what degree am I satisfied with my sexual identity, my sexual preferences, and my sexual behavior? How do I handle my sexual needs and wants?

My Strengths

_____

_____

_____

My Soft Spots

_____

_____

_____

G. RELATIONSHIPS, FAMILY. What are my deeper commitments like? How do I relate to family and relatives, however defined? How do I feel about the quality of my family or friendship-circle life?

My Strengths

_____

_____

_____

My Soft Spots

_____

_____

_____

H. CAREER. What is the place of work in my life? How do I feel about the way I am preparing myself for a career or the career I am currently pursuing? What do I get out of work? What am I like in the workplace? How does the workplace affect me? What impact do I have there?

My Strengths

_____

_____

_____

My Soft Spots

_____

_____

_____

I. INVESTMENT IN THE WIDER COMMUNITY. How big is my world? How do I invest myself in the world outside of friends, work, and the family? What is my neighborhood or community like? What kind of concerns do I have about community, civic, political, social issues? In what ways am I optimistic about the world? In what ways am I cynical?

My Strengths

_____

_____

_____

My Soft Spots

_____

_____

_____

J. LEISURE. What do I do with my free time? Do I feel that I have sufficient free time? How do I use my leisure? What do I get out of it? In what social settings do I spend my free time?

My Strengths

_____

_____

_____

My Soft Spots

_____

_____

_____

2. Once you have chosen three areas you think need some attention, jot down words, ideas, and sentences that relate to both your strengths and soft spots in these areas. Remember that an unused strength is really a soft spot, but a soft spot with potential.

EXERCISE 6.2: SELF-CHALLENGE REGARDING DEVELOPMENTAL TASKS

In this exercise we revisit the developmental areas in Exercise 6.1, but now from the perspective of self-challenge.

1. Review the three developmental "soft spots" you identified in Exercise 6.1.
2. Challenge whatever blind spots you might have in these areas and come up with one or two new perspectives in each area. Ask yourself: Where am I at currently in this developmental area? Where would I like to be? What is getting in the way of where I am and where I want to be?
3. Outline the kinds of actions these new perspectives might drive: What would you need to do in the short-term and long-term to get where you want to be?

Example. Jonathan, a 22-year-old who has just received his undergraduate degree with a major in psychology, had this to say:

Developmental areas: "I chose identity and investment in the wider community."
New perspective: "There is a huge difference between identity and what I now see as individualism. I think I've been on the selfish, me-first, what's-in-it-for-me track. I think little about the wider community and belonging to it. Now I'm about to join that community."
Action implications: "First of all, I have to clear up in my mind the difference between knowing who I am, what I stand for, and where I'm going versus my 'me-first' attitudes. Second, I'd like to begin to take a critical look at the messages the society of which I am a part has been screaming at me through music, movies, television, peer interaction, the internet, social media — the whole package. A lot of the messages that bombard me could be influencing me to remain an adolescent, but I don't want to remain an adolescent. I can't afford to remain an adolescent. Who would want to hire me!"

Now explore the developmental areas you have chosen for yourself.

First developmental area: Where am I?

_____

New perspectives: Where would I like to be? What is getting in the way of my being there?

_____

_____

_____

Link to action: What would I need to do in the short-term and long-term to get to where I want to be?

_____

_____

_____

63

_____

_____

_____

Second developmental area: Where am I?

_____

New perspectives: Where would I like to be? What is getting in the way of being there?

_____

_____

Link to action: What would I need to do in the short-term and long-term to get to where I want to be?

_____

_____

_____

_____

_____

_____

Share what you have learned with a partner from your training group. How clear are the issues? How concrete and realistic are the possible actions?

EXERCISE 6.3: IDENTIFYING DIFFERENT AREAS NEEDING CHALLENGE

Challenge focuses on dysfunctional mindsets, patterns of emotional expression, and behavior, whether internal or external. There are various ways in which clients need to be helped to challenge themselves in order to develop the kinds of new perspectives that lead to constructive problem-managing and opportunity-developing action. In this exercise you are asked to do the following:

1. Read the case and determine in what area and in what way this client might benefit from an invitation to self-challenge.
2. Sketch out briefly what some helpful new perspectives might look like.
3. Indicate what kind of constructive actions might flow from the new perspective.
4. Share your observations with a learning partner. Note the similarities and the differences among your suggestions. Discuss how you might proceed with each client. Discuss how invitations to self-challenge should be formulated and delivered.

Example: Keisha, a new counselor who has been working in a hospital setting for a number of months, has begun to confide in one of her colleagues who has worked in health-care facilities for about seven years. Keisha has intimated, however tentatively, that she feels that some of the medical doctors tend to dismiss her because she is new, because she is a counselor and not a medical practitioner, and because she is a woman. One doctor has been particularly nasty, even though he masks his abusiveness under his brand of "humor." One day her colleague says to her, "Don't take that stuff. Tell 'em what you think!" Keisha replies: "That will only make them worse. I think it more important to stand up for my profession by just being who I am and helping patients as much as possible. Their meanness is a punishment in itself. Anyway, it's a game that doctors play with everyone else in this hospital. That kind of thing has been going on forever. It's not such a big deal anyway."

What mindsets and behavior might be challenged here? Under the guise of "reasonableness," Keisha could be into excuse making. "This is the way it is and the way it will always be" seems to be her stance. Furthermore, Keisha says nothing about the possible impact of hospital politics on both staff and patients. **What would some helpful new perspectives look like?** Keisha might be helped to see that accepting the status quo goes counter to the kind of professionalism that should characterize the hospital and that she prides herself in. She may also be helped to see that the hospital's caste system might interfere with team approaches to helping patients.
What actions might such new perspectives lead to? Keisha might bring the core issues before the hospital senate, she might quietly lobby some of her colleagues to see what kind of consensus there is, she might talk to the especially abusive doctor privately and let him know how she feels, she might confide in one of the doctors who seems to be free of these prejudices in order to see what course of action she might follow, and so forth.

Now we turn to a range of clients. It goes without saying that the best way of doing this exercise is through actual interaction with these clients. At this stage, however, you are being asked to do some educated guessing.

1. Gabrielle and Pedro have tried unsuccessfully to have children. Doctors have examined both of them and now offer little hope even with new medical techniques. They have both been seeing a counselor, but in this session Gabrielle, who is much less reconciled to their fate than Pedro, is seeing the counselor alone. She says, "It's just not fair. Doctors talk about infertility as a clinical phenomenon, not a human reality. Pedro and I love one another. We want to have children. We'd make very good parents. We've done everything the doctors have told us to do, and still nothing. Pedro and I have to find the right hospital and the right doctors. We don't want to be told that adoption is the only possibility left."

What mindsets, behavior, and emotional expression might be challenged here?

_____

_____

_____

What would some helpful new perspectives look like?

_____

_____

_____

What actions might such a perspective lead to?

_____

_____

_____

2. Lynn, married with three teenage children, lost all the family's savings in a gambling spree. Under a lot of pressure from both his family and his boss, he started attending Gamblers Anonymous meetings. He seemed to recover, that is, he stopped betting on horses and ball games. A couple of years went by and Lynn stopped going to the GA meetings because he "no longer needed them." He even got a better job and was recovering financially quite well. But his wife began to notice that he was on the phone a great deal with his broker. She confronted him and he reluctantly agreed to a session with one of the friends he made at GA. He says, "She's worried that I'm gambling again. You know, it's really just the opposite. When I was gambling I was financially irresponsible. I bet our future on horses and ball games. But now I'm taking a very active part in creating our financial future. Every financial planner will tell you that investing in the market is central to sound financial planning. I'm a doer. I'm taking a very active role."

What mindsets, behavior, and emotional expression might be challenged here?

_____

_____

_____

What would some helpful new perspectives look like?

_____

_____

_____

What actions might such a perspective lead to?

_____

_____

_____

3. Stefan, a refugee who had been brutalized by a political regime in his native country, has been seeing a counselor in a center that specializes in helping victims of torture. He has been in the country for two years. He has a decent job. Even though he is now secure, at least in some sense of that term, he has found it very difficult to establish relationships with other refugees, with members of the immigrant community, or with native-born Americans. He intimates that he is quite lonely, but dismisses loneliness as "inconsequential" when the counselor brings it up. In one session, he says: "Let's not talk about my so-called loneliness when the world is filled with tragic loneliness. The loneliness that brutality creates, now that's something that counts. I fill my days quite well. When it is time, I'll seek out others, but I need people who can see the world as I see it. As it really is."

66

What mindsets, behavior, and emotional expression might be challenged here?

_____

_____

_____

What would some helpful new perspectives look like?

_____

_____

_____

What actions might such a perspective lead to?

_____

_____

_____

CHALLENGING NORMATIVE DISHONESTIES

Most of us face a variety of self-defeating dishonesties in our lives. We all allow ourselves, to a greater or lesser extent, to become victims of our own prejudices, smoke screens, distortions, and self-deceptions. Some of these normative dishonesties may have originated in lived experiences throughout our lives. These normative dishonesties may keep us away from facing some difficult challenges in our lives.

EXERCISE 6.4: CHALLENGING NORMATIVE DISHONESTIES IN ONE'S OWN LIFE

In this exercise you are asked to confront some of the ordinary ways in which we can be dishonest with ourselves and others. You are asked, as usual, to focus on the kind of dishonesties that might affect the quality of your helping or the quality of your membership in the training group.

Example 1. In this example a trainee confronts his need to control situations. She says, "I am very controlling in my relationships with others. For instance, in social situations I manipulate people into doing what I want to do. I do this as subtly as possible. I find out what everyone wants to do and then I use one against the other, and a little gentle persuasion, to steer people in the direction in which I want to go. In the training sessions I try to get people to talk about problems that are of interest to me. I even use empathic responses and probes to steer people in directions I might find interesting. All this is so much a part of my style that usually I don't even notice it. I see this as selfish, but yet I experience little guilt about it."

Example 2. This trainee confronts his need for approval from others. He says, "Most people see me as a 'nice' person. Part of this I like, but part of it is a smoke screen. Being nice is my best defense against harshness and criticism from others. I'm cooperative. I compliment others easily. I'm not cynical or sarcastic. I've gotten to enjoy this kind of being 'nice.' I find it rewarding. But it also means that I seldom talk about ideas that might offend others. My feedback to others in the group is almost always positive. I let others give feedback on mistakes. Outside the group I steer clear of controversial conversations. But I'm beginning to feel very bland."

Now confront two of your own "dishonesties," which, if dealt with, will help you be a more effective trainee and counselor. In the description section, be as specific as you can. As in the examples, describe specific experiences, behaviors, feelings, points of view, and decisions. Give brief examples.

Issue # 1

_____

_____

Describe your "dishonesties" and their possible impact on your role as helper.

_____

_____

_____

_____

_____

What should you do about this?

_____

_____

_____

Issue # 2.

_____

_____

Describe your "dishonesties" and their possible impact on your role as helper.

_____

_____

_____

_____

_____

What should you do about this?

_____

_____

BLIND SPOTS

Interestingly enough, when we are asked to take a look at our blind spots, we quickly begin to see what they are. Our "blindness" is cured. But most people don't ordinarily ask themselves, "What are my blind spots?" Read the section on blinds spots in Chapter 6 before doing these exercises.

EXERCISE 6.5: EXPLORING YOUR OWN BLIND SPOTS

We all have blind spots, but some are more damaging than others. In these exercises, try to focus on blind spots that may interfere with your competence as a helper.

1. Name a problem situation and an opportunity-development situation in your life which you did not address or did not address as well as you might have because of blind spots.
2. Review the following two examples and then move on to real situations in your own life.

Problem-Focused Example: Talitha came from a very strict family. Growing up was not at all unpleasant for her because she easily took to developing the kind of self-discipline that was expected of her. She and her two brothers studied hard, did their share of household work, attended church, and volunteered in the community. Brothers and sister got along well and cooperated to get things done. She grew up believing that if everyone didn't live this way, they *should*. At school and in the community she tended to become friends with like-minded young people. For the most part they avoided the "nonsense" that went on in school and in the community. She was pretty much unaware of what the world was really like. Her definition of "normal" was very restricted. At the end of high school she decided to get a job for a year or two before moving on to college. She got a job at a large retailer. The store she worked in anchored a suburban mall. At the store she met all sorts of young people, both coworkers and customers. Because so many of them did not seem to live up to her standards, she felt disorganized and frustrated. She got into a number of arguments with other workers and even with younger customers. On the verge of being fired, she quit. At home she became listless and sullen.

What blind spots might she have had and what possible part do you think they played in the difficulties she was experiencing?

_____

_____

_____

_____

Opportunity-Focused Example: Craig, a single man, retired on a modest company pension when he was 62. He also opted for the reduced social security pension which was still available for 62-year olds. These two sources of income enabled him to live modestly but comfortably. He owned the condominium in which he lived. Craig was an "avoider." Whenever there were problems at work, when people got in his hair, he daydreamed about how "great" retirement would be. He did little to prepare psychologically for retirement. Within a month he missed the social life at work and also the intellectual challenges of his job. He realized that he was still comparatively young. He lived in a city with a lot of amenities. His health was good. But three months after retiring, surrounded by opportunities, he was miserable.

What part did blind spots possibly play in his predicament?

_____

_____

_____

_____

Now focus on your own blind spots. It is difficult sometimes to recognize these blind spots. However, when looking back at situations we can sometimes see these blind spots.

Describe a problem situation in your own life you managed poorly because of blind spots.

_____

_____

_____

_____

Describe an unused opportunity in your own life you managed poorly because of blind spots.

_____

_____

_____

_____

_____

EXERCISE 6.6: HELPING OTHERS IDENTIFY AND DEAL WITH BLIND SPOTS

In this exercise you are asked to search your past and present relationships and interactions with others—relatives, friends, teachers, acquaintances, coworkers, and so forth—in order learn from the blind spots you have observed in them. This exercise deals with different levels of unawareness and tendencies to distort the world instead of seeing it as it is. Review the "Degrees of Awareness" section in Chapter 6 before doing this exercise. You are looking for blind spots that have caused or are now causing problems for the person. Blind spots deal with ways of thinking, modes of emotional expression, behavior, or a combination of all of these.

1. **Simple unawareness example**. Beth seems totally unaware of her failure to control the behavior of her two small children. This annoys most of her friends and is not in the best interest of the children. She misses the indirect "messages" that others send her.

Describe a case of simple unawareness from your experience.

_____

_____

_____

Describe the consequences of the blind spot.

_____

_____

_____

What could you do or have done to help the person become aware?

_____

_____

_____

2. **Failure to think things through example**. Cheryl and Chris get into trouble because they buy a house they like with an interest-only mortgage without considering the comparative price of real estate in the neighborhood, the state of the real estate market, the state of the economy, interests rates, the likelihood of their wanting to move later on, and so forth. Now they sit with an "under water" mortgage facing the threat of foreclosure.

Describe a case of failing to think things through.

_____

_____

_____

Describe the possible or actual consequences.

_____

_____

_____

What could you do or have done to help the person become aware?

_____

_____

_____

3. **Self-deception example.** Rebecca is deceiving herself when she says that she can stop using drugs without changes in her social life even though she hangs around with a group of people who are serious drug users.

Describe a case of self-deception.

_____

_____

_____

Describe the possible or actual consequences.

_____

_____

_____

What could you do or have done to help the person challenge his or her self-deception?

_____

_____

_____

4. **Choosing to stay in the dark example**. Lisa every once in a while picks up hints that her husband is dissatisfied with their relationship. Both are in their mid-30s and have full-time jobs. She notes the hints at the time they happen, but then puts them out of her mind. She does not want to deal with it. She also refuses to think about any kind of possible linkage among the various incidents.

Describe a case of choosing to stay in the dark.

_____

_____

_____

Describe the possible or actual consequences.

_____

_____

_____

What could you do or have done to help the person challenge his or her avoidance?

_____

_____

_____

5. **Knowing, not caring, and ignoring possible consequences example**. Fernando, who does not like his boss, lets her know in a variety of not-too-subtle ways. He knows that this annoys her, but in the back of his mind thinks that no single incident merits any kind of retaliation. His coworkers watch this little drama. Fernando knows that others are watching and prides himself with getting away with it.

Describe a case of knowing, not caring, ignoring possible consequences.

_____

_____

_____

Describe the possible or actual consequences.

_____

_____

_____

What could you do or have done to help the person challenge his or her behavior?

_____

_____

_____

SPECIFIC SKILLS FOR HELPING CLIENTS ENGAGE IN SELF CHALLENGE

Specific challenging skills, as outlined in Chapter 6 of *The Skilled Helper*, include sharing advanced empathic responses, information sharing, helper self-disclosure, suggestions, recommendations, confrontation, and encouragement. The purpose of these skills is to help clients get in touch with their blind spots and develop the kind of new perspectives or behavioral insights needed to complete the clarification of a problem situation or opportunity and to move on to developing possibilities for a better future, setting problem-managing goals, developing strategies, and moving to action. That is, challenging skills serve the entire helping process.

SHARING ADVANCED EMPATHIC RESPONSES

Advanced empathy, described most simply, means sharing educated "hunches" about clients and their overt and covert experiences, behaviors, and feelings that you think will help them see their problems and concerns more clearly and help them move on to developing new scenarios, setting goals, and acting.

Hunches should be based on your experience with your clients—what is happening in their lives, their behaviors and emotions, their points of view, the decisions they have made or are making, and their intended courses of action—both within the helping sessions themselves and in their day-to-day lives. Base your hunches on your relationship with your clients. Be hesitant to base your hunches on "deep" and speculative psychological theories. Be aware of the experiential and behavioral clues on which your hunches are based. In other words, know where your hunches come from and share them judiciously.

73

EXERCISE 6.7: ADVANCED ACCURATE EMPATHY—HUNCHES ABOUT YOURSELF

One way to get an experiential feeling for advanced empathy is to explore *at two levels* some situation or issue in your own life that you would like to understand more clearly. One level of understanding could be called the surface or immediate level. The second could be called a deeper or more thoughtful level. Often enough reality is found at the more thoughtful level.

Read the following examples.

Example 1: A man, 25 years old, in a counselor training program is having his ups and downs in the training group. He is having second thoughts about his ability and willingness to get close to others.

Level-1 understanding: "I like people and I show this by my willingness to work hard with them. For instance, in this group I see myself as a hard worker. I listen to others carefully and I try to respond carefully. I see myself as a very active member of this group. I take the initiative in contacting others. I like working with the people here."

Below-the-surface understanding: "If I look closer at what I'm doing here, I realize that underneath my hardworking and competent exterior, I am uncomfortable. I come to these sessions with more doubts than I have admitted, even to myself. My hunch is that I have some hesitation about closeness to others. I am afraid that both here and in a couple of relationships outside the group someone is going to ask me for more than I want to give. This keeps me on edge here and in a couple of relationships outside."

Example 2: A woman, 33 years old, in a counselor training group, sees that her experience in the group is making her explore her attitude toward herself. It might not be as positive as she thought. She sees this as something that could interfere with her effectiveness as a counselor.

Level-1 understanding: "I like myself. I base this on the fact that I seem to relate freely to others. There are a number of things I like specifically about myself. I'm fairly bright. And I think I can use my intelligence to work with others as a helper. I'm demanding of myself, but I don't place unreasonable demands on others."

Below-the-surface understanding: "If I look more closely at myself, I see that when I work hard it is because I feel I have to. My hunch is that "I-have-to" counts more in my motivation than "I-want-to." I get pleasure out of working hard, but it also keeps me from feeling guilty. If I don't work hard enough as I define the term, then I can feel guilty or down on myself. I am beginning to feel that there is too much of the I-must-be-a-perfect-person in me. This leads to my judging both myself and others more harshly than I should."

1. Choose an issue, topic, situation, or relationship that you have been investigating and that you would like to understand more fully with a view to taking some kind of action on it. Try to choose issues that might affect the quality of your counseling.
2. Briefly describe the issue, as in the examples.
3. Then give a "surface-level" description of the issue.
4. Next, share some hunch you have about yourself that relates to that issue, a hunch that "goes below the surface," as it were, but don't try to "psych yourself out." This will help you get in touch with possible blind spots. Try to develop a new perspective on yourself and that issue, one that might help you see the issue more clearly so that you might begin to think of how you might act on it.
5. Share your insights with your learning partner. Discuss the action implications of these insights.

74

Issue # 1.

_____

_____

_____

Level-1 understanding.

_____

_____

_____

_____

Below-the-surface understanding.

_____

_____

_____

_____

_____

Issue # 2.

_____

_____

Level-1 understanding.

_____

_____

_____

Below-the-surface understanding.

_____

_____

_____

_____

_____

EXERCISE 6.8: ADVANCED VERSUS BASIC EMPATHIC RESPONSES

1. In this exercise, assume that the helper and the client have established a good working relationship, that the client's concerns have been explored from his or her perspective, and that the client needs to challenge himself or herself to see the problem situation from some new perspective or to act on the insights that have been developed.
2. In each instance, imagine the client speaking directly to you.
3. First respond to what the client has just said with a basic empathic response.
4. Next, formulate one or two hunches about this person's experiences, behaviors, feelings, point of view, decision, or intended course of action—hunches that, when shared, would help promote the kind of new perspectives that drive problem-managing or opportunity-developing action. Use the client's statement and context to formulate your hunches. Ask yourself: "On what clues am I basing this hunch?"
5. Finally, respond with some form of advanced empathy, that is, share some hunch that you believe will be useful for him or her.

Example: A man, 48 years old, who is a husband and father, is exploring the poor relationships he has with his wife and children. In general, he feels that he is the victim, that his family is not treating him right (that is, like many clients, he emphasizes his experience rather than his behavior). He has not yet examined the implications of the ways he behaves toward his family. At this point he is talking about his pride in being a breadwinner. He says: "I work really hard to be a good provider. In fact, I'm more than a provider. I travel a lot and don't really like traveling. But this means that I can provide not just the basics but little luxuries. You know, nice holidays and things like that. But I think I'm more appreciated at work than at home. They see how hard I have to work. Often enough I have to spend hours in my home-office to prepare for my trips. For all this I get a pretty grumpy group at times."

Basic empathic response. "It's irritating when your own family doesn't seem to appreciate what you're doing for them, the sacrifices you're making to give them a better life."
Hunch. The family wants a husband and father, not just a breadwinner or gift-giver. He has unilaterally made a decision to work long hours in order to be the kind of provider he wants to be.
Advanced empathic response. "It might be possible that their 'grumpiness' is not a sign of ingratitude but frustration because you've chosen not to be around very much."

Now try your hand at the following cases.

1. Margaret, a first-year engineering graduate student, has been exploring her disappointment with herself and with her performance in school. Her father is a successful engineer, but has not pressured his daughter to follow in his footsteps. Margaret has explored with her counselor such issues as her dislike for the school and for some of the teachers. She says: "I just don't have much enthusiasm. My grades are just okay, maybe even a little below par. I know I could do better if I wanted to. I don't know why my disappointment with the school and some of the faculty members can get to me so much. It's not like me. Ever since I can remember—even in primary school, when I didn't have any idea what an engineer was— I've wanted to be an engineer. Theoretically, I should be as happy as a lark because I'm in a graduate school with a good reputation, but I'm not."

Basic empathic response.

_____

_____

_____

76

Your hunch and your reason for it.

_____

_____

_____

_____

Advanced empathic response.

_____

_____

_____

2. This man, now 64 years old, retired early from work when he was 60. He and his wife wanted to take full advantage of their "golden" years. But his wife died a year after he retired. At the urging of friends he has finally come to a counselor. He has been exploring some of the problems his retirement has created for him. His two married sons live with their families in other cities. In the counseling sessions he has been alternately dealing the theme of loss and the theme of redefining his golden years. He says: "I seldom see the kids. I enjoy them and their families a lot when they do come. I get along real well with their wives. But, since my wife has been gone, I don't make the effort I should to make it happen. I have a standing invitation from the boys and just recently I've decided I'm going to get off my sofa and start living again. I won't kid you; it will be bittersweet. I dread those times when I'll want to turn to her and enjoy the moment and she won't be there. I don't want my boys to see their father shattered and I sure as hell don't want to see pity in their eyes."

Basic empathic response.

_____

_____

_____

Your hunch and your reason for it.

_____

_____

_____

_____

Advanced empathic response.

_____

_____

INFORMATION SHARING

As noted in the text, sometimes clients do not get a clear picture of a problem situation or manage it effectively because they lack information needed for clarity and action. Information can provide clients with some of the new perspectives they need to see problem situations as manageable or to spot and embrace unused opportunities. Giving clients problem-clarifying information or, better, helping them find it themselves, is not, of course, the same as advice giving or preaching.

EXERCISE 6.9: INFORMATION LEADING TO NEW PERSPECTIVES AND ACTION

In this exercise you are asked to consider what kind of information you might give or help clients obtain which would enable them to see their problem situations or opportunities more clearly. Information can, somewhat artificially, be divided into two kinds: (a) information that helps clients understand their difficulties better and (b) information about what actions they might take.

Example: Tim was a bright, personable young man. During college he was hospitalized after taking a drug overdose during a bout of depression. He spent six months as an in-patient. He was assigned to "milieu therapy," an amorphous mixture of work and recreation designed more to keep patients busy than to help them grapple with their problems and engage in constructive change. He was given drugs for his depression, seen occasionally by a psychiatrist, and assigned to a therapy group that proved to be quite aimless. After leaving the hospital, his confidence shattered, he left college and got involved with a variety of low-paying, part-time jobs. He finally finished college by going to night school, but he avoided full-time jobs for fear of being asked about his past. Buried inside him was the thought, "I have this terrible secret that I have to keep from everyone." A friend talked him into taking a college-sponsored communication-skills course one summer. The psychologist running the program, noting Tim's rather substantial natural talents together with his self-effacing ways, remarked to him one day, "I wonder what kind of ambitions you have." In an instant Tim realized that he had buried all thoughts of ambition. After all, he didn't "deserve" to be ambitious. Tim, instinctively trusting him, divulged the "terrible secret" about his hospitalization for the first time. With some encouragement from the psychologist, Tim decided to try counseling to address this realization further.

Tim and his counselor, Rick, had a number of meetings over the course of a year. In some of the early sessions Rick provided him with information that proved challenging in a number of ways. For instance, when it came to employment, the counselor helped Tim find out that:

- he was more intelligent and talented than he realized and, therefore, that he was underemployed;
- that his hospitalization was quite different from, say, a felony conviction;
- deep background checks were not required for the kinds of jobs that Tim might apply for;
- privacy laws often protect prospective employees from damaging disclosures;
- enlightened employers look benignly on developmental crises during a prospect's adolescence;
- the job market was strong and growing stronger, so that people with Tim's skills and potential were in high demand.

All this challenged Tim to look at himself in a different light, that is, as a potential winner instead of a loser, and to move more aggressively into job hunting.

In the following cases, you are not asked to be an information expert. Rather, from a lay person's or a common-sense point of view, you are asked to indicate what kinds of information you believe might help the client understand and manage the problem situation more clearly. What blind spots do you think the client might have? How do you think information might help? In what ways would the information be challenging?

1. Point out the blind spots the client might have.
2. Indicate what information could help the client get some new perspectives and move to action.

1. A man, 26 years old, has just been sentenced to five years in prison on a felony burglary charge. He is talking to a chaplain-counselor who has worked for the past ten years at the prison to which the man has been assigned. The man is somewhat cavalier about spending time in the prison. He spends a lot of time looking for ways to overturn his conviction and is preoccupied with the possibility of early parole. His main regret is that he was caught.

What blind spots might the client have?

_____

_____

_____

What information might help this client develop new perspectives?

_____

_____

_____

_____

In what way might this information be challenging for the client?

_____

_____

_____

_____

2. A 58-year-old woman has endured an almost year-long struggle to find out what has been sapping her energy. Her doctors first thought she was depressed and started her on medication but she saw little improvement and she had to contend with the side effects. Time passed and she lived in uncertainty. Recently, her doctors arrived at a diagnosis—chronic fatigue syndrome. When they told her, the woman's reaction took them a little by surprise. While she was full of questions about what it all meant, still she

seemed relieved and eager to get on with whatever would be required. She said it was such a relief to finally know where she stood.

What blind spots might the client have?

_____

_____

_____

What information might help this client develop new perspectives?

_____

_____

_____

_____

In what way might this information be challenging for the client?

_____

_____

_____

_____

_____

HELPER SELF-DISCLOSURE

Although helpers should be *ready* to make disclosures about themselves that would help their clients understand their problem situations more clearly, they should do so only if such disclosures do not upset their clients or distract their clients from the work they are doing. Read the text on helper self-disclosure before doing this exercise.

EXERCISE 6.10: EXPERIENCES OF MINE THAT MIGHT BE HELPFUL TO OTHERS

In this exercise you are asked to review some problems in living or unused opportunities that you feel you have managed or are managing successfully. Indicate what you might share about yourself that would help a client with a similar problem situation. That is, what might you share of yourself that would help the client move forward in the problem-managing process?

Example 1: "In the past I have been an expert in feeling sorry for myself whenever I had to face any kind of difficulty. I know very well the rewards of seeing myself as victim. I used to fantasize myself as victim as a form of daydreaming or recreation. I think many clients get mired down in their problems because they let themselves feel sorry for themselves the way I did. I think I can spot this tendency in others. When I see this happening, I think I could share brief examples from my own experience and then ask clients to see if what I was doing squares with what they see themselves doing now."

80

Example 2: "I have been addicted to a number of things in my life and I see a common pattern in different kinds of addiction. For instance, I have been addicted to alcohol, to cigarettes, and to sleeping pills. I have also been addicted to people. By this I mean that at times in my life I have been a very dependent person and I found the same kind of symptoms in dependency that I did in addiction. I know a lot about the fear of letting go and the pain of withdrawal. I think I could share some of this in ways that would not accuse or frighten clients or distract them from their own concerns."

1. List two areas in which you feel you have something to share that might help clients who have problems in living that are similar to your own. Just briefly indicate the area.
2. Next, indicate what you might share.
3. Share these with a learning partner. Give and get feedback on the appropriateness and usefulness of the disclosures. Discuss the conditions under which you would share what you have written.

Area # 1.

_____

_____

What in this area might you share, if appropriate?

_____

_____

_____

_____

Area # 2.

_____

_____

What in this area might you share, if appropriate?

_____

_____

_____

EXERCISE 6.11: PUTTING IT ALL TOGETHER IN A HELPING SESSION

1. Choose one of the problem situations and/or unused opportunities you have been discussing with yourself and your learning partners. Make sure it has substance and there is still work to do.
2. Write out a summary of where things stand in your personal case. Provide whatever detail is necessary. Share this with the learning partner who will be your helper.
3. Have a half-hour session with your designated helper. See what progress the two of you can make. Video the session.

4. The learning-partner/helper uses whatever communication skills he or she believes necessary to help his or her colleague/client make progress.
5. At the end of the half hour do a collaborative debrief of the session using both the video and dialogue.
6. Switch roles and repeat the exercise.

Chapter 7

HELPER SELF-CHALLENGE

Inviting our clients to challenge themselves is a deeply personal and difficult process. Invitations should be framed within a caring, genuine, and empathetic therapeutic relationship. Further, inviting clients to self-challenge can be enhanced by fully understanding clients' experiences, promoting responsibility, and focusing on outcomes. The following exercises are aimed at enhancing your ability to invite clients to self-challenge. You need to challenge yourself before inviting others to challenge themselves. Read "The Guidelines for Effective Invitations to Self-Challenge" before doing these exercises.

EXERCISE 7.1: EARNING THE RIGHT TO INVITE CLIENTS TO CHALLENGE THEMSELVES

One of the principal ways you put yourself in the position of inviting clients to challenge themselves is developing and maintaining a decent collaborative relationship with the client. Reread what is said about an effective therapeutic relationship in Chapters 1 and 2 and earning the right to invite clients to challenge themselves in Chapter 7. Then evaluate how effective you have been in developing your relationship skills.

1. What have you done both inside the training group and outside to become better at building relationships?

_____

_____

_____

_____

2. What about you gives you the "right" to invite clients to challenge themselves?

_____

_____

_____

_____

3. Share what you have written with a learning partner. Try to find one who knows you well. See if you get any new insights from this discussion.

EXERCISE 7.2: INVITATIONS TO SELF-CHALLENGE THAT PROVIDE "CHOICE STRUCTURE"

Reread the parts of Chapters 5 and 7 dealing with nudging, choice structure, and decision making. When clients face difficult decisions, your job is to help them face up to these decisions. *How* you provide

83

"choice structure" and "nudge" them toward life-enhancing decisions is critical. The following cases involve, directly or indirectly, invitations to self-challenge. Evaluate them by discussing your reactions with a learning partner.

Case 1. This client is in dire financial straits. He has been discussing the possibility of filing for bankruptcy with his financial counselor. At one point the counselor says, "I know that you want to do everything possible to avoid bankruptcy. If it is inevitable, I think that you might want to choose it rather than be forced into it. I wondering if this is a good time to discuss both the upside and the downside of bankruptcy. It might put you in a better position to make a choice."

Discuss your reaction to this invitation with a learning partner. Upside? Downside?

Case 2. This client has been talked into an abortion by both her parents and her boyfriend. Since then she has manifested many of the symptoms of PTSD. "I know that you're really feeling awful about the abortion. It might help to explore what's driving your feelings. You can't keep refusing to discuss why you feel so bad. Do you think you caved in to pressure? Or is it something else? If you don't talk about what's making you feel so bad, you won't get anywhere. But I'm not sure you're ready to do that or not. How can I help you?"

Discuss your reaction to this invitation with a learning partner. Upside? Downside?

Case 3. This client sees his brief affair with another woman as one of the worst mistakes of his life. He has kept it to himself, but it is haunting him. "I can understand why you want to tell your wife about the affair. You really want to 'come clean' as a way of putting the affair behind you. You see it as a way of being honest, not just with her, but with yourself. But you do seem hesitant to tell her. It might be useful to explore your hesitancy, especially because you don't want to cause her any further anguish."

Discuss your reaction to this invitation with a learning partner. Upside? Downside?

EXERCISE 7.3: EFFECTIVE VERSUS INEFFECTIVE CHALLENGE

The way in which you challenge clients is extremely important. You need to challenge others in such a way that they will *respond* rather than *react* to your invitations.

In this exercise, you are asked to practice on yourself. It goes without saying that you should not practice ineffective challenging on others, even colleagues in your training group.

1. Choose an area in which you feel that you need to challenge yourself. It can relate either to a problem situation or some unused resource or opportunity.
2. Write out a self-challenge statement in which you violate the principles of effective challenging outlined in Chapter 6 & 7.
3. Then write a self-challenge statement that embodies these principles.

Example. This therapy trainee is challenging himself on a certain lack of discipline in his life.

Poor invitation to self-challenge: "You're disorganized and lazy. Your room and your desk are continually messy and your excuse is that you are so busy. But that's a lame excuse. You waited until the end of the course to do the required papers and therefore their quality is poor. In some ways it is worse in your interpersonal life. You're always late. Others have to wait for you. It's a way of saying you're more important than others. You're just inconsiderate. Since all of this is so ingrained in you, you're not going to change—unless something drastic happens."

Effective invitation to self-challenge: "You do reasonably well in school and your social life is quite decent. However, there is the possibility that both could be even more satisfying. At school you tend to put things off, sometimes to the point that rushing affects the quality of your work. For instance, end-of-semester papers. Since you pride yourself on giving your best, putting things off like that is not fair to yourself. You keep telling yourself it's time to get better organized, but you need to come up with a plan for doing so. What would some of the elements of such a plan be?"

4. Share both forms of self-challenge with a learning partner and discuss. The flaws in the poor self-challenge could be subtle or quite evident. Identifying what makes the "appropriate" challenge effective is important.

EXERCISE 7.4: CHALLENGING YOUR OWN UNUSED STRENGTHS

Inviting clients to challenge unused or partially used strengths rather than weaknesses is one of the principles of effective challenge. In this exercise you are asked to challenge yourself with respect to your own unused or underused strengths and resources, especially those that would help make you a better therapist.

1. Briefly identify some problem situation or unused opportunity.
2. As in the example, indicate how some unused or underused strength or strengths you have could be applied to the management of the problem situation or unused opportunity.
3. In addition, indicate some actions you might take to make use of underused strengths.

Example 1. Katrina, a trainee in her early 20s, is concerned about bouts of anxiety. She has led a rather sheltered life and now realizes that she needs to "break out" in a number of ways if she is to be an effective counselor. The counseling program has put her in touch with all sorts of people, and this is anxiety-provoking. She lists some of the strengths she has that can help her overcome her anxiety.

Description of underused strengths or resources and some possible actions: "I'm bright. I know that a great deal of my anxiety comes from fear of the unknown. I'm intellectually adventuresome. I pursue new ideas. Perhaps this can help me be more adventuresome in seeking new experiences involving relationships."

Actions I can take to develop and use these resources: "The best way to dissipate my fears is to face up to situations that cause them. New ideas don't kill me. I bet new experiences won't either. People find me easy to talk to. This can help me form friendships. My fears have kept me from developing friendships. However, developing more relationships is one of the best ways of preparing to be with clients."

4. Now apply the same procedure to one problem situation and one unused opportunity.

1. Problem situation.

_____

_____

85

Underused strengths as applied to the problem situation.

_____

_____

_____

Actions you could take to make use of this underused resource in this problem situation.

_____

_____

_____

2. Unused opportunity.

_____

_____

Underused strengths as applied to the unused opportunity.

_____

_____

_____

Actions you could take to make use of this underused resource to develop this opportunity.

_____

_____

EXERCISE 7.5: TENTATIVENESS IN THE USE OF CHALLENGING SKILLS

As noted in the text, invitations to self-challenge are usually more effective if they do not sound like accusations. Therefore, in challenging clients, don't accuse them, but don't be so tentative that the force of the challenge is lost.

1. Return to Exercise 6.8 on advanced empathy in Chapter Six.
2. With a learning partner, review the responses you wrote there in terms of tentativeness.
3. Improve responses that would benefit from more or less or better expressed tentativeness.
4. Share your redone responses with a learning partner and provide mutual feedback.

DEALING WITH RELUCTANCE AND RESISTANCE

In order to recognize reluctance and resistance in clients, it helps to first be able to recognize the same tendencies within yourself and learn how to manage them in your own life. These exercises help you look at your own reluctance and resistance.

EXERCISE 7.5: MY OWN RELUCTANCE IN EMBRACING DEVELOPMENTAL CHALLENGES

Since living more effectively requires hard work, is sometimes painful, and entails risk, all of us express reluctance from time to time. This exercise targets your own reluctance to become more than you are.

1. Review the developmental challenges in your life you identified in EXERCISE 6-1.
2. Identify three areas or ways in which you have been reluctant to grow or change. Spell them out in some detail. Note the difference between reluctance and resistance.

First area of reluctance.

_____

_____

_____

Second area of reluctance.

_____

_____

_____

Third area of reluctance.

_____

_____

_____

3. Have your learning partner pick one of these areas, one that he or she thinks might stand in the way of being an effective helper. Have a 15 minute counseling session with him or her. During the session find one or more opportunities to invite him or her to self-challenge. Video it.
4. Use the video in debriefing the session with your learning partner. Get feedback on your communication style and your ability to invite clients to challenge themselves.
5. Switch roles and repeat the exercise.

EXERCISE 7.6: IDENTIFYING AREAS OF RELUCTANCE RELATED TO BECOMING AN EXCELLENT PROFESSIONAL

The assumption is that you want to be more than a run-of-the-mill professional. However, most professions, including psychotherapy, are of their very nature very demanding. Therefore, it is not uncommon to feel some reluctance to dive into the work needed to become a top-notch professional. This is not about competition. It is about excellence. In this exercise you are asked to take a good look at your own areas of reluctance.

87

Example. Michaela, 19, a first-year student in clinical psychology, has this to say about developing a sense of responsibility: "The more I learn about the world, the more I see how comparatively easy life has been for me. Everything has been given to me. I'm a product of the American dream. I had an easy time in high school. College was a bit more demanding, but I eased by. But the first months of graduate school have been jarring. Becoming a really good professional is very demanding. As I look down the road I see that grad school more accurately reflects the real world. Without getting into useless guilt trips, I realize I'm spoiled. I also realize that old habits do not die easily. I still expect things to be handed to me on a platter. I'm reluctant to face up to the realities of imposed schedules, competition, demanding work, and budgets. It is very difficult for me to accept that some of my learning is going to come from making mistakes, being challenged, and having to do things over. And research seems to be such a tedious occupation. Am I in the right place?"

Now identify three areas of your own reluctance to face the demands of becoming a first-class professional.

First area of reluctance.

_____

_____

_____

Second area of reluctance.

_____

_____

_____

Third area of reluctance.

_____

_____

_____

3. As you share these instances of personal reluctance with a learning partner, see if you can identify any underlying themes that run through all three areas.

_____

_____

_____

4. Choose one of the areas or the theme that runs through all three and indicate what you might do in order to overcome your reluctance.

_____

_____

88

_____

_____

_____

_____

EXERCISE 7.7: MY OWN EXPERIENCE OF RESISTANCE

Recall that resistance is a reaction to someone's trying to force you to change when you don't want to. The other person may or may not be pressuring you, but you *feel* pressured. You may even think that the other person has a point, but the fact that he or she is *telling* you what to do causes you to react negatively rather than respond constructively.

1. Recall two instances when you resisted growth because you felt you were being forced into it.
2. Indicate how you could have transformed that negative experience into a positive one for yourself.

Example. Manfred, a 24-year-old graduate student in social work, recalls being badgered by a former girlfriend: "Elise was out to reform me. It's not that I was not in need of reform during my college years. But the way she went about it turned me off. For instance, I drank too much. But she lectured me in private. Then she embarrassed me in front of my friends—her way of getting my attention. Before going out to major events like the homecoming dance, she laid down rules and made me promise to keep them. Otherwise she wouldn't go out with me. Things like that."

When asked how that negative experience could have been turned into a positive one, he had this to say: "The substance of what she was saying actually made sense. But I would have done better if she had backed off a bit, quite a bit at times. For instance, instead of laying down rules to prevent disasters, she could have quietly left the scene if they did occur. If she had said that she was no longer having fun and was going home and then just did it a couple of times, I think that would have been a real wake-up call for me. I could have said all of this to her, but I never did. I just reacted."

One instance of resistance in your own life:

_____

_____

_____

Indicate how that negative experience could have become a positive one for you.

_____

_____

_____

_____

89

A second instance of resistance in your own life:

_____

_____

_____

Indicate how that negative experience could have become a positive one for you.

_____

_____

_____

_____

_____

EXERCISE 7.8: YOUR ROLE IN CAUSING CLIENTS TO RESIST

Resistance in clients is often prompted by real or perceived coercion on the part of the helper. As a helper, you may not think that you are putting any undue pressure on a client, but he or she might feel that you are. That is, you don't intend to be coercive but nevertheless you come across that way. For example, let's assume that you are very open about yourself. That's the way you grew up. However, when you place a demand on others for higher levels of self-disclosure than they are ready for, they may clam up. Therefore, there is much to be gained from knowing what aspects of your own style might come across to others as subtly, or not so subtly, coercive.

Example: Marisol, 42, is an experienced counselor working in a health-care facility. Recently, she transferred within the hospital from the emergency room where she handled individuals and families in crisis to the oncology unit. She talks about how her emergency-room style has caused problems in the oncology unit: "Down in the ER we had to work fast and I got good at making things happen. Now I'm in oncology and I'm getting on people's nerves. I feel like I'm out of synch. I want to help both staff and patients make decisions but our timetables are all different. I'm moving fast, you know, the way I did in the emergency room. And I want people to move at my pace. I'm scaring some people. Others are grateful for my assertiveness and candor. I need to tailor my style to the unit, to the different situations, and to different people. I have to pay close attention to what people need and then pace myself."

1. Jot down some aspects of your interpersonal style that might be seen as coercive by others. If you see none, don't invent any. Just say so.

Coercive aspects of your style.

_____

_____

_____

Changes that would help.

_____

_____

_____

2. Discuss with your partner what aspects of your helping style could be a problem for at least some clients. Finally, talk about ways of changing or softening your style.

PART III
THE SKILLED HELPER PROBLEM-MANAGEMENT AND OPPORTUNITY-DEVELOPMENT APPROACH TO HELPING

Chapter 8

AN OVERVIEW OF THE PROBLEM-MANAGEMENT PROCESS

Chapter 1 provided a broad picture of the problem-management and opportunity-development process. Part III provides a detailed picture of this process, which serves as an integrative framework for all the key ingredients of successful therapy. Chapter 8 provides a more detailed overview of the problem-management process, but it is still just that—an overview. The details follow in Chapters 9-14. If possible, do exercise 8.1 before reading Chapter 8 or completing the other exercises in this chapter.

EXERCISE 8.1: WHAT DO PEOPLE THINK COUNSELING INVOLVES?

As we have seen, one of your jobs as therapists is to explain what therapy is about and the approach you are taking. Getting clients on board the problem-management process is critical. It helps, then, to know what might be in the client's mind as he or she arrives for the first session. This exercise is designed to give you some sense of how helping, counseling, or therapy (whatever the name used) is seen by the "public." This exercise does not pretend to be a scientific investigation.

1. Interview three or four friends, relatives, or colleagues. Ask them what they think counseling is.
2. Get more than just a definition. Using your communication skills, help them expand on whatever definition or description they provide.
3. Write a summary of the main facets in their definitions and descriptions.
4. Meet with two or three of your fellow learners and share what you've discovered.
5. What range of definitions/descriptions of counseling emerges from your discussion? What are the themes? What are the variations?
6. Finally, discuss the importance of sharing with clients what your approach to counseling is, what the helper's role and responsibilities are, and what the client's role and responsibilities are.

EXERCISE 8.2: EXPLAINING THE BASIC TERMINOLOGY

You need to understand and be ready to explain to others two terms used throughout the problem-management process. They are "stage" and the "tasks" within the stages. Understanding these two terms is essential for understanding the kind of client-focused flexibility that permeates the problem-management process. Do this exercise with a learning partner.

1. Have a discussion with your learning partner about what the term "stage" means and does not mean. If you disagree in any way, be ready to explain both the agreements and the disagreements to others. Finally, write out your common understanding (the elements you agree on) of the term "stage."

"Stage" means:

_____

_____

_____

_____

_____

2. Repeat the above for the term "task."

"Task" means:

_____

_____

_____

_____

3. Share your findings with another group. Finally, the instructor will take up the issue with the entire training group. The outcome is a shared understanding of both these terms.

4. Why is a clear understanding of these terms important?

_____

_____

_____

EXERCISE 8.3: WHAT KIND OF PROBLEM-MANAGER AND OPPORTUNITY-DEVELOPER AM I?—A SELF-ASSESSMENT

As a counselor, you are going to be helping clients manage problem situations and develop unused or underused opportunities. It would be odd if you were not using these same skills in managing your own life. Here is an opportunity to use the problem-management process or framework as a self-assessment tool. Helpers can and should become better problem managers throughout their lives. Rate each of following on a scale from 1-7 (with 7 as a high score). As mentioned before, when self-rating, push yourself to be honest.

Stage I:-Task-A Behaviors
- _____ I spot problem situations as they begin to develop.
- _____ I tend to address issues directly and immediately.
- _____ I act on the "prevention is better than cure" principle.
- _____ I'm always on the watch for life-enhancing opportunities.
- _____ I analyze problem situations clearly; I quickly grasp what's going on.
- _____ I quickly analyze the potential of any given opportunity.
- _____ I apply these behaviors to the rest of problem management—goal setting, strategy development, and implementation.

Name one behavior you would like to be better at.

_____

_____

Stage I: Task-B Behaviors
- _____ I am open to getting feedback from others.
- _____ I find ways of getting in touch with my blind spots
- _____ I am open to exploring my blind spots with others.
- _____ I translate blind spots into useful, life-enhancing new perspectives.
- _____ I understand that I can have blind spots at any stage or task of the helping process.
- _____ I am a vigilant person.

Name one behavior you would like to be better at.

_____

_____

Stage I: Task-C Behaviors
- _____ I know how to separate the important issues of life from the trivial.
- _____ I know the difference between what is critical and what is merely useful.
- _____ In both problem management and opportunity development I focus on the bigger issues of life.
- _____ I do not let myself become a victim of the trivial things of life.

Name one behavior you would like to be better at.

_____

_____

Stage II: Task-A Behaviors
- _____ I'm open to problem-managing and opportunity-developing possibilities.
- _____ The psychology of hope is important for me.
- _____ I brainstorm about the future.
- _____ The concept of "possible selves" is important for me.
- _____ I look for ways of increasing my creativity.

Name one behavior you would like to be better at.

_____

_____

Stage II: Task B-Behaviors
- _____ Goals play an important role in my life.
- _____ Even though I am goal-driven, I am still flexible.
- _____ My goals have the kind of focus and clarity needed to drive action.
- _____ I appreciate all kinds of goals—emerging, adaptive, and coping.
- _____ I tailor goals to the kind of problem situation or opportunity at hand.

Name one behavior you would like to be better at.

_____

_____

94

Stage II: Task C-Behaviors

- _____ I have a practical understanding of the dynamics of incentives, commitment, and motivation.
- _____ The goals I set are both useful and in some way appealing even when they are difficult.
- _____ I take my commitments—both to myself and to others—seriously.

Name one behavior you would like to be better at.

_____

_____

Stage-III Behaviors

- _____ I know that there are usually a number of paths to a goal.
- _____ I explore these paths diligently.
- _____ I choose strategies that fit my style and the circumstances.
- _____ Whenever required, I turn the strategies I choose into a step-by-step plan.
- _____ My plans are living realities, not just words on a page.

Name one behavior you would like to be better at.

_____

_____

Implementation Behavior

- _____ I am a doer, not just a dreamer.
- _____ As soon as I start to think about a problem situation or an opportunity, I begin engaging in little actions that get me moving toward more substantial outcomes.
- _____ The stages and tasks outlined above make me think of things I can do.
- _____ I am open to changing my cognitive behavior, my external behavior, and/or the ways I express my emotions.
- _____ My actions are usually focused, not just actions for the sake of action.

Name one behavior you would like to be better at.

_____

_____

General Problem Management Behavior

- _____ The behaviors outlined above constitute a mentality, a way of approaching life.
- _____ The behaviors outlined are often implicit rather than explicit.
- _____ The framework is in my bones; it is part of my lifestyle.

All in all, what kind of problem manager are you? Where do your strengths lie? Your weaknesses?

EXERCISE 8.4: PREPARING TO TELL YOUR STORY—PROBLEM SITUATIONS

As mentioned earlier, the counselor training program is an opportunity for you to examine many different aspects of your life and to make changes that will help you become an effective therapist. All helpers have problems or issues that could lessen their effectiveness. Knowing what yours are is an important part of training. You have already completed some exercises that were designed to help you spot strengths and weaknesses in your life. Here is one more self-exploration exercise as you move into learning and practicing the problem-management process in detail. The following sentence-completion exercise will help you to choose issues that you would like to and are willing to discuss. Do these sentence-completion exercises quickly.

1. One of my biggest problems is
2. I'm quite concerned about
3. Something I fail to do that gets me into trouble is
4. The social setting of life I find most troublesome is
5. The most frequent negative feelings in my life are
6. These negative feelings take place when
7. The person I have most trouble with is
8. What I find most troublesome in this relationship is
9. Life would be better if
10. I tend to shortchange myself when I
11. I don't cope very well with
12. I get anxious when
13. A value I fail to put into practice is
14. I'm afraid to
15. I wish I
16. I wish I didn't
17. What others dislike most about me is
18. I don't seem to have the skills I need in order to
19. A problem that keeps coming back is
20. If I could change just one thing in myself it would be

Once you have finished, place a check-mark next to the issues you might be willing to discuss with a friend, partner, or in the training group. Then circle the checked issues you believe are most closely related to becoming an effective helper. Finally, with a learning partner, discuss the items you have both checked and circled.

EXERCISE 8.5: PREPARING TO TELL YOUR STORY—UNUSED OPPORTUNITIES

This sentence-completion exercise mirrors the preceding one but deals with unused or underused strengths and opportunities rather than problems. Undeveloped strengths and opportunities can affect the quality of your helping.

1. I could be better at
2. Those who know me know that, when I want to, I can
3. I've always wanted to
4. I regret that I haven't
5. When I'm at my best I
6. I'm glad when I
7. Those who know me know that I can
8. A value that I try hard to practice is
9. When I'm at my best with people I
10. I can't always count on myself to
11. Something I'm handling better this year than last is
12. If I were managing my life better I would
13. A recent problem I haven't handled as well as I might is
14. I have the courage to
15. I aspire to
16. I think that I have the guts to

96

17. An example of some unfinished business I have is
18. When I think of my maturity I
19. One way in which I could be more dependable is
20. I communicate most effectively with others when

Once you have finished, place a check-mark next to the unused opportunities you might be willing to discuss with a friend, partner, or in the training groups. Then circle the checked issues you believe are most closely related to becoming an effective helper. Finally, discuss the items that you have both checked and circled with a learning partner.

EXERCISE 8.6: FLEXIBILITY OF THE PROBLEM-MANAGEMENT FRAMEWORK IN ACTION

As noted in Chapter 8 of the text, the problem-management framework is intended to be flexible. This flexibility is an acknowledgement that making progress on a problem can unfold in a variety of ways, depending on the values and preferences of the client. If you have a solid understanding of the terms "stage" and "task," it will become clear how flexibly you can use them.

1. What is meant by the "sequential logic" of the stages and tasks of the problem-management process?

_____

_____

2. How does the "clinical use" of the stages and tasks of the problem-management process take precedence over its "sequential logic"?

_____

_____

3. Explain this statement: Clients can begin their stories anywhere they want in the "geography" of helping.

_____

_____

4. Explain this statement: Within therapy, clients can move to whatever stage or task they think will be helpful.

_____

_____

5. Explain this statement: Throughout therapy, therapists can suggest that the client move to a stage or task of the problem-management process that the therapist believes will help the client make progress—doing so, however, in collaboration with the client.

_____

_____

EXERCISE 8.7: STARTING POINTS AND FLEXIBILITY

When clients tell their stories, they start anywhere within the "geography" of helping. It is your job to know what their starting point is, to follow their logic, and to help them engage in whatever stages and tasks that will help them achieve the outcomes they are looking for. Name the starting point for each of the following cases.

1. Read the case, answer the questions, and check out your answers with a learning partner.

Case 1. Jessica looks very harried. She sits down but does not seem to know where to start. Finally she says, "It's just not working. I've done just about everything the bank's financial 'counselor' asked me to do. I've made a budget. I've cut back on my credit card use. I'm living very frugally. I buy just necessities. And still they won't do anything to help me stave off foreclosure proceedings. I'm at my wit's end!"

The client's starting point

_____

_____

How would you proceed?

_____

_____

Case 2. The client is a sailor who has just been released from captivity. He spent three weeks in the custody of pirates who captured his ship. He has been back home for two weeks. He speaks very hesitatingly as he says, "This has been one of the worst times of my life. I felt that my life was in danger every minute I was there. I thought being freed would take care of everything. But I'm still a mess. I can't sleep. I thought it would be great to get back to my family, but, to tell the truth, I haven't been easy to live with. My whole life has changed.

The client's starting point

_____

_____

How would you proceed?

_____

_____

Case 3. This client has just got out of jail. As a pedophile, his name is on the sexual predator list. He is a mandated client. Getting post-imprisonment therapy was a requirement for his release. He says, "I just can't go back to jail. Ever! But if I'm honest with myself, I can say that I never want to offend again. Part of me really means that for a whole variety of reasons. But you've seen a lot of guys like me. You know and I know that the urges just don't go away. That's the other side of me. What do people like me do?"

98

The client's starting point

_____

_____

How would you proceed?

_____

_____

Case 4. This client has been out of work for 18 months. His job search has been very frustrating. He says, "Eighteen months and not even a nibble. Forty years old and nothing! Now this week I get two job offers and it's got me all twisted up. I've got a degree in civil engineering. I've been offered a job by a real estate developer. The pay is quite decent. It would help me put my finances back in order. But the company is new and who knows what's going to happen in commercial real estate over the next few years. The second offer I got by networking with a couple of friends of mine. It's with the city. The pay isn't that good, but the are some tradeoffs. My assumption is that job security would be better. But is it security in a sort of dead end job? And there is a pension scheme. But who knows what's going to happen with government pension schemes? Two job offers. I should be deliriously happy, but I'm in turmoil."

The client's starting point

_____

_____

How would you proceed?

_____

_____

2. How much do your answers differ from those of your learning partner? How can you go about reconciling the differences?

EXERCISE 8.8: USING CLIENT FEEDBACK

Regularly monitoring the progress of treatment, the quality of the helping relationship, and the value of each session is a key ingredient of successful therapy. Then, if anything goes wrong, you can address it immediately and make the needed changes. Below, you are given the opportunity to practice asking for feedback from clients who have sought your help. For each of the case examples provided, do the following:

1. Write down some ideas you think would be helpful to address the following three areas:

A. Progress being made on the identified problem. Select a way that is comfortable for you to discuss with the client what progress (or the lack thereof) that he or she is making (some helpers use a rating scale to describe progress, while others ask open-ended question such as "How far along do you think you are in managing the problem situation?").

99

B. The quality and usefulness of each session and the helping relationship itself. Select a way that is comfortable for you to ask how the client feels about how you are working on the problem together (How satisfied are you with the way we are working on your concerns? How has this session gone?).

C. Making use of feedback. Identify what you might change as a result of the feedback you receive from the client.

Example: Samirah, a beginning counselor, has been working with Garett for three sessions. Garett sought help in order to decide whether he wants to leave his marriage of five years or stay and try to work on it. He has a 10-month-old daughter but has become increasingly unhappy with his marriage. His wife had a brief affair 3 years ago, and he has been unable or has refused to forgive her. He was going to leave the marriage but she became pregnant and now he is confused about what he should do. He is thinking of staying because of the child although he believes she got pregnant to save the marriage. Samirah has been focused on the concept of forgiveness. At the beginning of the fourth session, Samirah asks Garett for feedback:

A. Progress in Managing the Problem Situation

Samirah: Garett, I wanted to check in and ask about your progress on making a decision. How much closer do you feel like you are to making a decision compared to our first session?

Garett: I feel like I have made some progress. I didn't realize how angry I was at her and how trapped I feel. I can see the reasons for wanting to leave versus staying more clearly. The next likely goal for me will be to develop a plan and get the courage to leave.

B. Helpfulness of the Relationship and the Sessions

Samirah: Well, overall, how do you think we're doing together?

Garett: I am lot more comfortable with you now, but it's still hard work. I really believe that you have my best interests at heart and I know you won't try to force me into any decision.

Samirah: How do you think today's session went?

Garett: I squirmed when you invited me to talk about what I think might be going on inside my wife. I think it was your way of maybe helping me to find more constructive ways of talking with her. But what you did was fair. I want to be fair, too, even though I'm still angry.

Samirah: Is there anything you would change about how we're working together?

Garett: We've focused a lot on forgiveness and that has felt less helpful. I have forgiven a lot in our marriage and I am usually the one in relationships who just sucks it up. I go along to get along, if you know what I mean. Maybe it's time for me to stand up for myself and acknowledge that what I feel matters.

C. Making Use of the Feedback

Samirah suggested that in the next session she might role play his wife and Garett could experiment ways of expressing his anger and hurt—not as ways of retaliating, but as ways that would facilitate progress in decision making and moving away from "swallowing his feelings" to expressing them both honestly and constructively.

2. Choose one of the following examples and, like the Samirah-Garett case, write a scenario depicting how a request for feedback might go and how you as a therapist would make use of the feedback. Deal with progress (or the lack thereof) being made, the helpfulness of the session, the quality of the relationship, and making use of the feedback. Use your imagination in developing the case.

Case 1. Federico has seen Ellen, a 20-year-old African American female, for five sessions at a university counseling center. Ellen sought therapy because she felt depressed and is tired of feeling "ugly and fat." Federico has talked about exercise as one way to feel better and address her concerns with her weight.

Ellen has reluctantly agreed but has not been very talkative and rarely makes eye contact. She has not reported any improvement or differences in previous sessions.

Case 2. Terry, a 42-year-old White male, has had one session with his drug and alcohol counselor Pam on his long-standing drinking problem. He sought treatment because he is tired of living alone and living a "dead end life." He wants to quit drinking and go back to school. Terry played professional baseball after signing a contract out of high school; he got injured and lost his dream of playing in the major leagues. He is now motivated by a new dream—being a high school teacher and coach. Pam has primarily focused on listening to and understanding his story and has started to ask about his drinking behaviors and what triggers his drinking to excess. Terry has been sober for a week and seems excited about continuing treatment.

3. Share your scenario with a learning partner. Provide each other with constructive feedback.

Chapter 9

STAGE I-A:
HELP CLIENTS TELL THEIR STORIES

Clients come to helpers because they need help in managing their lives more effectively. The communication skills needed to help clients tell their stories are covered in Part II of the text. Chapter 9 lays out the principles for using these skills. The three interrelated "tasks" of Stage I illustrate three ways in which counselors can help clients tell their stories. This is not an information gathering stage. Rather the goal of Stage I is to help client tell their stories in such a way as to come to a fuller and more realistic understanding of themselves, their problem situations, and their unused opportunities. There are three interrelated tasks in Stage I:

Task A: Stories. Help clients tell their stories, share their points of view, explore their decisions, and clarify what they intend to do together with the emotions involved.
Task B: Real Stories. Help clients identify and move beyond blind spots to new perspectives that will help them manage their problem situations and opportunities more effectively.
Task C: Right Stories. Help clients work on issues that will most likely make a difference in their lives. Helping is a collaborative search for value for the client.

Chapter 9 focuses on Task A, helping clients tell their stories as clearly as possible. Since these three tasks are interrelated and apply to all the stages and tasks of the helping process, clarity is always needed. As indicated in *The Skilled Helper*, the principles embedded in these three tasks are not restricted to Stage I for the following reasons. First of all, clients don't tell their full stories at the beginning of the helping process. Often the story "leaks out" over time. Second, new perspectives can be helpful in any stage or task of the helping process. New perspectives are useful in choosing goals, developing strategies for implementing goals, and in the implementation process itself. Third, value in the broadest sense deals with the "economics" of helping. Choosing the right problem or opportunity to work on is just the beginning. Choosing the right goals, strategies, and resources for implementation is also part of the picture. "Right" means right for this client in this situation. Read Chapter 9 in the text before doing the exercises in this section.

EXERCISE 9.1: HELPING ONE ANOTHER TELL YOUR STORIES

In this exercise you have the opportunity of playing three roles successively: the client, the helper, and the observer.

1. Form groups of three.
2. In each group there are three roles: client, helper, and observer. You will play all three roles. Quickly decide who will play what role to begin.
3. Before the dialogue between client and helper begins, the trainee in the client role gives a brief summary of the problem situation or unused opportunity he or she is going to explore. Choose a developmental issue discussed in Chapter 6 of these exercises or any other issue you are willing to explore. Remember the rules outlined in the introduction to this manual. *No one should be forced to talk about themselves; they should do so freely.*

Example: Enrico, the trainee playing the role of client, gives the following summary: "I'm going to discuss a problem I'm having with my parents. I'm an only child and they simply won't let go. Don't get me wrong. They're very nice about it. But I'm 21. We're not a wealthy family. So, for the time being, I have to live at home. Also I believe that becoming my own person is directly related to becoming an effective helper."

1. The helper begins by saying: "Against that background, Enrico, what would you like to focus on today?"
2. Then client and helper engage in a helping dialogue. The counselor helps the client tell his or her story clearly and in useful detail.
3. After about 10 minutes or so the observer, in timekeeper mode, stops the dialogue.
4. The client gives the helper feedback on how effectively he or she has aided the storytelling process. Feedback should cover communication skills—such as nonverbal behavior, empathic responses, open-ended versus closed-ended questions, other probes or "nudges," and invitations to self-challenge. Feedback should also focus on the "Guidelines for Helping Clients Tell Their Stories" covered in Chapter 9.
5. Because giving feedback to your fellow learners is an important part of the training program, review the section in the Introduction on guidelines for giving effective feedback.
6. Then the observer shares his or her observations.
7. The process continues until each member has had the opportunity to play each role.
8. After each group member has played each role, discuss what you have learned. What did helpers do that enabled clients to speak more easily and clearly?

EXERCISE 9.2: UNDERSTANDING THE SEVERITY OF THE PROBLEM
It is important to gauge the severity of clients' problems from the onset. This exercise builds on exercise 9.1.

1. Read the section on problem severity in Chapter 9.
2. Each counselor should have a second five-minute session with his or her client moving more deeply into the problem situation discussed as part of EXERCISE 9.1.
3. Using the criteria from Chapter 9, rate the severity of your client's problem. 1-7 _____ .
4. Share your rating with the client and the reasons behind it.
5. Discuss the reasons behind your rating through a dialogue with the client.
6. Get feedback from the observer on how useful this exercise has been.
7. Repeat the exercise until each participant has had the opportunity to play each role
8. End up with a three-way dialogue on the importance of assessing the severity of clients' problems. What impact on your approach to clients should such assessments have?

EXERCISE 9.3: REVIEWING YOUR OWN PAST

Consider some problem situation or unused opportunity you are currently dealing with. Think through the possible past roots of the current situation.

1. On a separate sheet of paper jot down ways you think the past has had some influence on the present problem situation.

Example. Here is what one trainee named Keith had to say to his internship supervisor: "In my culture, treating guests and even strangers with respect and even indulgence was a pervasive expectation. As I review my family history I believe that some relatives, friends, and strangers took advantage of this cultural prescription. Even when we suspected that this was happening, the cultural imperative took precedence. We seldom called anyone's 'game.' Although to a lesser extent, I think that this norm or value still influences me significantly. Even when clients are evasive or play games, I am hesitant to help them take a closer look at what they are doing. These strangers are still my 'guests.' In some sense of the term I 'indulge' them. But I'm not doing them any service by acting this way."

2. Now do the same for a problem situation.

What is the current problem situation?

_____

_____

_____

In what ways is some past experience possibly influencing it?

_____

_____

_____

_____

What do you need to do to manage it?

_____

_____

_____

_____

3. Do the same for some unused opportunity.
4. Debrief both problem situation and unused opportunity with a learning partner in terms of talking productively about the past.

EXERCISE 9.4: HELPING CLIENTS TALK PRODUCTIVELY ABOUT THE PAST

Clients will of necessity talk about what has happened to them in the past. In some cases the client uses the past to add depth to their story or to supply needed context. However, at other times clients talk about the past without any effort to make a link to what is presently happening in their lives. Read the section in *The Skilled Helper* on how to make talking about the past productive.

1. Pick a partner to do this exercise either inside or outside the classroom. In this exercise listen to your partner discuss a past event in his or her life.
2. Next, help your partner to draw from the past event some implications for the present. Base your invitation on the principles outlined in Chapter 9.
3. When you have finished discuss the session with your partner. How did you help your partner connect the past to the present? What else could you have done to help your partner see the implications of the past for the present?
4. Start by indicating what you would do if you were the counselor in the following case.

104

Case: Kirk, who is 28, is about to finish a doctoral program in clinical psychology. His problem situation revolves around his relationships with women. He has just started dating someone seriously. He is reflecting on a past relationship that didn't work out. He says to you: "This happened about three years ago. I guess I didn't realize it then, but I was in a relationship with a really great woman, one of the best I will ever know. We fell for each other and everything was great. Then we had this fight about how to relate to our respective families. They were quite different from each other. I told her that we should keep our distance. She took an almost opposite stand. I kept pushing. I guess I made it almost impossible for her. I was really stubborn. Angry, too. I told her she sounded like my mom. The fact that she had a strained relationship with my mom didn't help. Well, after that, out of spite, I guess, I began seeing other women. Of course, she found out. I might have salvaged it even then if I had gone to her and said what I really felt. Instead I just began to spend more time with my drinking buddies and played the field. But now I've recovered enough to start dating someone seriously."

What would your approach to Kirk be?

_____

_____

What would you do to help him link the past to the present?

_____

_____

Now have a real counseling session with one of your learning partners who will start by talking about his or her past. Afterwards debrief the session in terms of the principles related to talking about the past productively.

EXERCISE 9.5: CLARIFYING KEY ISSUES

Remember that helping clients clarify issues pertains to every stage and task of the helping process. In this exercise each participant, when in the role of the client, discusses a problem situation or unused opportunity that needs clarification. As clients talk about their stories, the goal for change can become clearer to both client and counselor. The purpose of this exercise is to help make the goals for counseling more explicit.

1. When you are in the client role, first provide some overall context for what you are going to discuss.
2. Next present a *vague* problem-managing or opportunity-developing *goal*. Your counselor's job is to help you clarify that goal.
3. Spend about ten minutes or so pursuing clarity through dialogue. Use all the communications skills outlined in Part II to help your client achieve the kind of clarity needed to move forward in the problem-management process. Video the session.
4. At the end of 10 minutes check to see if the client has the kind of clarity to move forward. If not, continue for another five minutes. If the client feels satisfied, stop and debrief the sessions with the help of the video.
5. Finally, switch roles. This time the client starts by summarizing some problem situation and a clear goal he or she has set in order to manage the problem situation. However, the client is not sure what he or she should do next. That is, the client has only a few vague ideas about how to achieve the goal. Help him or her to clear up the vagueness.

Example. Let's take the example of a real client. Anastasia is in jail on a charge of manslaughter. Her background is not pretty: poverty, undereducated, drug use, overweight, and more. Because of her erratic driving in a borrowed car one evening, she killed a man. It was not a hit-and-run. In fact, she is deeply sorry for what happened. All she can say is, "It just happened. A thousand things were going through my mind. I got lost in myself and hit him. I wasn't high." Her trial is coming up and she has no idea what to do. During a session with a counselor, she says, "I want the right me to be there. I'm not a bad person. The right me has to be there." By "there" she means at the trial.

The counselor takes her vague goal, "the right me at the trial," and helps Anastasia clarify it. In the end that means that Anastasia wants to appear contrite, because she is. While often she is disheveled, she wants to look as decent as possible at the trial, "because I am decent." She wants to be able to answer questions reasonably well. That, too, is part of "the right me." She clams up when confronted. Helping Anastasia clarify her goal proves to be invaluable. The counselor goes on to help her find ways to achieve the goal, which is really a self-presentation package. What Anastasia instinctively wanted was not a phony package, but the real one. In the end, she was convicted of a lesser charge and given probation.

Remember, the first client starts with a vague goal. When roles are switched, the second client starts with a clear goal but a vague plan.

EXERCISE 9.6: HELPING YOURSELF DISCOVER AND EXPLOIT YOUR UNUSED STRENGTHS AND RESOURCES

As you listen to clients tell their stories you may well note strengths and resources they have failed to use to manage the problem situations or unused opportunities they are discussing. You will add a great deal of value if you help them get in touch with relevant strengths and resources.

1. Think of one problem situation and one unused opportunity in which, using hindsight, you failed to use strengths and resources that were available to you.

Example. Trudy was job hunting, but unemployment was very high and jobs were hard to come by. It was more difficult for her because she did many different things after graduating—traveling to see foreign student friends and their families, getting involved in some church-related social service projects, and the like—so she was not a freshly minted graduate nor did she have an employment history. She sent her resume to many different Internet-based job search sites, such as monster.com. She also researched companies on the Internet and applied for job openings listed on their sites. In addition, she contacted a recruiting agency and had an initial interview with them. All of this led nowhere. However, there were two resources she failed to use. One was the alumnae association of the university she graduated from. It was renowned for its job finding prowess. She had not even joined the association or any of its subgroups. Contact through family, friends, and friends of friends constituted the other unused resource. When asked about these unused resources, she replied laconically, "I can do this by myself." She became depressed and saw a counselor. Fairly quickly, the counselor began to help her explore what might be behind her reluctance to network.

1. Problem situation.

_____

_____

What resources were available to you but remained unused?

_____

_____

_____

Describe how these resources might have made a difference.

_____

_____

_____

2. Unused opportunity.

_____

_____

What resources were available to you but remained unused?

_____

_____

Describe how these resources might have made a difference.

_____

_____

_____

EXERCISE 9.7: HELPING CLIENTS DISCOVER AND EXPLOIT UNUSED STRENGTHS AND RESOURCES

Think of someone you know fairly well who is involved in a problem situation, and who has both the strengths and resources to manage it but does not either recognize or use these strengths and resources. Also think of someone you know fairly well who has some unused opportunity that could enrich his or her life, together with the strengths and resources needed to pursue this opportunity, but fails to do so.

1. Start with the person who has a problem situation he or she is not managing very well. Answer the following questions.

Describe the nature of the problem situation.

_____

_____

_____

_____

107

Describe the unused strengths and resources that are relevant to the problem situation.

_____

_____

_____

_____

_____

2. Do the same thing for the person with the unused opportunity.
3. Share your cases with a learning partner and discuss how you would go about helping these people tap into these unused strengths and resources.

EXERCISE 9.8: LINKING STORYTELLING TO ACTION

As noted in the text, clients need to engage in "little" actions throughout the helping process that get them moving in the right direction even before formal goals and action strategies are established. These little actions are signs of clients' commitment to the process of constructive change. In this exercise you are asked to put yourself in the place of the client and come up with some possible actions that the client might take to move forward in some way. You are not going to tell the client what to do. But helping clients adopt an action orientation to their problem situations is central to helping.

1. Read each of the stories outlined below.
2. If you were the client, what are two common-sense actions you might consider taking at this stage in order to move forward? Even if "big" actions seem premature, what "little" actions might you take? Indicate the reason for each possible action.

Example. A seventh-grade boy talking to his father (all this is said in a halting voice and he keeps looking down): "Something happened yesterday that's bothering me a lot. I was looking out the window after school. It was late. I saw two of the guys, the bullies, beating up on one of my best friends. I was afraid to go down there. . . . A coward. . . . I didn't tell anyone, I didn't do anything."

One possible action: The boy might talk the incident through with his friend and perhaps apologize for letting him down.
Reason: To reestablish trust with his friend and to show basic decency. To clear his conscience.
Another possible action: The boy and his father might discuss how to handle similar situations in the future.
Reason: To learn something useful from this painful experience. To turn a problem into an opportunity.

Case 1. A young woman talking to a counselor in a center for battered women. She has been seen by other counselors on two different occasions: "This is the third time he's beaten me up. I didn't come before because I still can't believe it! We're married only a year. After we got married, he began ordering me around in ways he never did before we got married. He'd get furious if I questioned him. Then he began shoving me if I didn't do what he wanted fast or right. And I just let him do it! I just let him do it! (She breaks down and sobs.) And now three beatings in less than two months. What's happened? Oh what's happened?"

Two possible client actions and a reason for each.

_____

_____

_____

_____

_____

_____

Case 2. A man, 70, arrested for stealing funds from the company where he has worked for 25 years, talking to an assigned social worker. This is their second session: "To tell you the truth, it's probably a good thing I've been caught. I've been stealing on and off for the last five or six years. It's been a game. It soaked up my energies, my attention, distracted me from thinking about getting old. Now I'm saying to myself: 'You old fool, what are you running from?' You're probably thinking: 'It's about time, old guy.'"

Two possible client actions and a reason for each.

_____

_____

_____

_____

_____

_____

Case 3. A girl, 15, talking to a psychologist at a time when her parents are involved in a divorce case: "I still want to do something to help, but I can't. I just can't! They won't let me. When they would fight and get real mean and were screaming at each other, I'd run and try to get in between them. One or the other would push me away. They wouldn't pay any attention to me at all. They're still pushing me away. They don't care how I think or feel or what happens to me! My mother tells me that kids should stay out of things like this."

Two possible client actions and a reason for each.

_____

_____

109

_____

_____

_____

_____

_____

Case 4. A young man, 24, is talking to his mentor, a senior partner in the company. A department head has offered him a managerial job in her area. In this job he will be leading an important project. He says, "I didn't think this kind of opportunity would come so soon. But I've decided to say yes. I'm a bit worried, sure, but I figure I was asked because they think I can do the job. You know, just three years ago I was studying this stuff in school and now I'm going to have a budget, people reporting to me, and a chance to make a mark. I have a pretty clear idea about what I'm going to do when I get started next week. Most of all I want to get off on the right foot with everyone."

Two possible client actions and a reason for each.

_____

_____

_____

_____

_____

_____

_____

3. Share your findings with a learning partner and get feedback on the actions you propose and the reasoning behind them.

Chapter 10

STAGE I
TASK I-B: THE REAL STORY AND
TASK I-C: THE RIGHT STORY

This chapter has two sections. The first section addresses the work on client self-challenge, focusing on the quality of client participation and collaboration in the helping process. Helping clients challenge themselves is, in the end, of way of helping them add value to their lives. The first section also provides counselors with guidelines to help them challenge wisely. The second section deals with the third task of Stage I of the helping process. This task focuses on helping clients choose to works on issues that have substance to them, that is, issues that will make a difference in their lives. More broadly, this task as applied to all the stages and tasks of the helping process focuses on seeking substance and value throughout the change process.

TASK I-B: THE REAL STORY
FURTHER THOUGHTS ON INVITATIONS TO SELF-CHALLENGE

This section deals with helping clients challenge themselves to find value by participating as fully as possible in the helping process. Helping is, ideally, a collaborative venture. This section also deals with the wisdom-informed guidelines needed to challenge well.

ENCOURAGING CLIENT PARTICIPATION

Clients add value by owning and participating as fully as possible in the helping process. This section focuses on some of the challenges to engagement clients face. Even clients whose good will is beyond doubt can have trouble participating for a variety of reasons. First, clients may lack the skills, especially the communication skills, needed to participate fully. If this is the case, you can use your communication skills to help them overcome obstacles to participation. For instance, if Alex is having problems with expressing himself use probes to help "walk" him toward clarity. Second, clients do not participate fully because they do not understand what the helping process is or how it works. If this is the case find ways to help them understand the essentials of the helping process as suggested in Chapter 8 of *The Skilled Helper*. Third, clients are often reluctant to participate fully in the helping process because they are reluctant to change. In helping sessions, clients manifest reluctance in many, often covert, ways. They may talk about only safe or low-priority issues, seem unsure of what they want, benignly sabotage the helping process by being overly cooperative, set unrealistic goals and then use their unreality as an excuse for not moving forward, not work very hard at changing their behavior, and be slow to take responsibility for themselves. They may blame others or the social settings and systems of their lives for their troubles and play games with helpers. Reluctance admits of degrees; clients typically come "armored" against change to a greater or lesser degree. Make sure you become a partner with your clients in overcoming whatever form of reluctance they get mired in. Finally, clients fail to participate because they resist what they see as your heavy-handed approach to change. When clients resist, they are no longer partners but adversaries. Chapter 9 provides hints on to how to befriend a client's reluctance or resistance.

111

EXERCISE 10.1: HELPING CLIENTS OWN PROBLEMS AND UNUSED OPPORTUNITIES

The more fully clients take responsibility for their problem situations and unused opportunities, the more likely are they to try to do something about them. In this exercise you are asked to look at the ways that you and someone you know own, or fail to fully own, problem situations and/or unused opportunities.

Example. Sam, 75 years old, is addicted to painkillers. He uses over-the-counter drugs to get rid of even the slightest pain. Because he is getter older, these pains are now more frequent and so his use of drugs is increasing. What does Sam need to know and do in order to own this problem situation?

1. Review the problem situations and unused opportunities in your own life that you have identified in previous exercises.
2. Pick one problem situation that still persists.
3. Jot down the ways in which you are failing to fully own the problem.

_____

_____

_____

4. Indicate what you need to do in order to fully own the problem or unused opportunity and act on it.

_____

_____

_____

5. Repeat this process with respect to someone you know who does not own some problem situation enough to do something about it. What does this person need to do in order to move forward? How might you help him or her?

EXERCISE 10.2: INVITING CLIENTS TO STATE PROBLEMS AS SOLVABLE

Often enough clients present problems as unsolvable. Occasionally problems are unsolvable but more often clients have trouble, for one reason or another, in being able to identify potential solutions. One reason can be that they have made several unsuccessful attempts and feel there are no options, while another reason might simply be to avoid the responsibility of doing something about them. As a helper, your role is to empower people to utilize their own resources and not rely on you or others to fix their problems – unfortunately there is no professional magic we possess that will dispose of the problem. Remember, as you help clients to own their problems and to view them as solvable, use your developing counseling skills and avoid being critical and harsh.

Example. Monica, a single mother, is having difficulty controlling the self-destructive behavior of her teenage daughter. She says something like this: "Things were so different when you and I were young. Today society is drowning in permissiveness. Kids get away with things at school that would have gotten us expelled. Krystal (her daughter) is constantly telling me what other kids and other parents are doing. I just get overwhelmed. She sees me as just old-fashioned, out of it. I feel like I'm always swimming against the tide."

1. Give an empathic response to Monica.

_____

_____

_____

2. What could you do to help her restate the problem situation in more solvable terms? What would you say to her to invite her to do so?

_____

_____

_____

3. Do the same for one of your own persistent problems or unused opportunities. In what ways do you think of it, at least covertly, in unsolvable terms? Revisit the problem situation or unused opportunity using solvable language.

IMMEDIACY: EXPLORING YOUR RELATIONSHIP WITH A CLIENT

As noted in the text, your ability to deal directly with what is happening between you and your clients in the helping sessions is an important skill. **Relationship** immediacy refers to your ability to review the history and present status of your relationship with another person, including clients and the members of your training group. **Here-and-now** immediacy refers to your ability to deal with a particular situation that is affecting the ways in which you and another person are relating right now, at this very moment. Immediacy is a complex skill. It involves: (1) revealing how you are being affected by the other person, (2) exploring your own behavior toward the other person and its impact, (3) sharing hunches about your behavior toward him or her, (4) sharing hunches about his or her behavior toward you, (5) pointing out your own and the other's discrepancies, distortions, smoke screens, and the like, and (6) inviting the other person to explore the relationship with a view to developing a better working relationship—all through dialogue. For instance, if you see that a client is manifesting hostility toward you in subtle, hard-to-get-at ways, you may: (1) let the client know how you are being affected by what is happening in the relationship (that is, you share your experience), (2) explore how you might be contributing to the difficulty, (3) describe the client's behavior and share reasonable hunches about what is happening (challenge), and (4) invite the client to examine in a direct way what is happening in the relationship. Immediacy involves collaborative problem solving and opportunity development with respect to the relationship itself.

EXERCISE 10.3: RESPONDING TO SITUATIONS CALLING FOR IMMEDIACY

In this exercise a number of client-helper situations calling for some kind of immediacy on your part are described. You are asked to consider each situation and respond with some statement of immediacy. Consider the following example.

Situation. Tom, a 44-year-old Asian-American man, occasionally makes snide remarks either about the helping profession itself or some of the things that you do in your interactions with him. At times he is cooperative and takes responsibility for himself, but at other times he gets on edge and asks you to make decisions for him. He is not beyond comments such as, "Just tell me the best way for me to tell my boss that he's an idiot." He makes remarks about you personally at times, "I bet you've got a lot of friends." Or, on being invited to challenge himself, "You just won't let me alone, will you?"

Immediacy response. "Tom, let's stop a minute and explore what's happening between you and me in our sessions. . . . (Tom says, "Uh, oh, here we go!") . . . You take mild swipes at the counseling profession such as, 'I hear people are still trying to find out whether counseling works.' Or at me, like, 'Oh, oh, Mr. Counselor is getting a little hot under the collar.' I've ignored these remarks, but in ignoring them I've become a kind of accomplice. Sometimes we seem to be working like a team. And we get things done. Other times you ask me to make decisions for you — you know, the 'just-tell-me' approach. I've let myself get on edge with you and that's not helping us at all. . . . (Tom says, "You want to call my game, huh?") . . . Tom, I guess that I prefer that we not even play games with each other at all. Perhaps we could spend a little time re-setting our relationship."

1. Critique the approach this counselor takes in the example. What would you change?
2. Share your critique with a learning partner.
3. Consider the following situations and write out an immediacy response that helps the client challenge unhelpful perspectives and actions.
4. Share your responses with a learning partner and give feedback to each other. Together, come up with more effective immediacy responses.

1. **The situation.** The client is a person of the opposite sex. You have had several sessions with this client. It has become evident that the person is attracted to you and has begun to make thinly disguised overtures for more intimacy. The person finds you both socially and sexually attractive. Some of the overtures have mild sexual overtones.

Immediacy response.

_____

_____

_____

_____

_____

2. **The situation.** In the first session you and the client, a relatively successful businessman, 40, have discussed the issue of fees. At that time you mentioned that it is difficult for you to talk about money, but you finally settled on a fee at the modest end of the going rates. He told you that he thought that the fee was "more than fair." However, during the last few sessions he has been dropping hints about how expensive this venture is proving to be. He talks about getting finished as quickly as possible and intimates that is your responsibility. You, who thought that the money issue had been resolved, find it still very much alive.

Immediacy response.

_____

_____

_____

_____

_____

3. **The situation.** The client is a young woman, 22 years old, who is obliged to see you as part of being put on probation for a crime she committed. She is cooperative for a session or two and then becomes quite resistant. Her resistance takes the form of both subtle and not-too-subtle questioning of your competence, questioning the value of this kind of helping, coming late for sessions, and generally treating you like an unnecessary burden.

Immediacy response.

_____

_____

_____

_____

EXERCISE 10.4: IMMEDIACY WITH THE OTHER MEMBERS OF YOUR TRAINING GROUP

This exercise applies to members of an experiential training group. It could be called an immediacy "round robin." The exercise assumes that you have interacted for a number of weeks and have gotten to know one another fairly well.

1. If the group is large, divide up into subgroups of about four trainees per group.
2. Read the example below.
3. On separate paper, write out a statement of immediacy for each of the members of your group.
4. Imagine yourself in a face-to-face situation with each member successively. Deal with real issues pertaining to the training sessions, interactional style, and so forth.
5. In a round robin, share with each of the other members of the group the statement you have written for him or her. Obviously it would be better to speak it than read it.
6. The person listening to the immediacy statement should reply with an empathic response, making sure that he or she has heard the statement correctly.
7. Then listen to the immediacy statement the other person has for you and reply with an empathic response.

115

8. Finally, engage in a dialogue for a few minutes about the implications of the two statements for both your interpersonal style and for this relationship.

9. Continue with the round robin until each person has had the opportunity to share an immediacy statement and have a dialogue with every other member.

Example: Trainee A to Trainee B. "I notice that you and I have relatively little interaction in the group. You give me little feedback; I give you little feedback. It's almost as if there is some kind of conspiracy of non-interaction between us. I appreciate the way you participate in the group. For instance, the way you invite others to challenge themselves. You do it carefully but without any apology. I think I refrain from giving you feedback, at least negative feedback, because I don't want to alienate you. I do little to make contact with you. I have a hunch that you'd like to talk to me more than you do, but it's just a hunch. I'd like to hear your side of our story."

With a learning partner, identify the elements of immediacy (self-disclosure, challenge, invitation) in this example. Then move on to the exercise.

SECTION II.
STAGE I: TASK C
HELP CLIENTS WORK ON ISSUES THAT WILL
ADD VALUE TO THEIR LIVES

The exercises in Task C deal with helping clients work on issues that will make a difference in their lives. Counseling time is too precious to waste on issues that do not add real value to a client's life. Read the section "Task I-C: The Right Story" in Chapter 10 of *The Skilled Helper* before doing the exercises in this section.

EXERCISE 10.5: HELPING CLIENTS SCREEN PROBLEMS

Clients may need help in determining whether their issues are important enough to bring to a helper in the first place or what form of help is needed. For example, someone who seeks counseling to lose weight and improve his financial status may benefit more from seeing a nutritionist, a personal trainer, or a financial counselor. A helper has to determine if he or she is the right person at the right time for a particular client. This is called "screening."

1. Read these two case summaries with a view to discussing them with your fellow trainees.
2. Discuss these two cases in terms of the material in the text on screening. Consider these questions.

> How would you approach the woman in Case 1?
> Under what conditions would you be willing to work with her?
> How would you approach the man in Case 2?
> In what general ways does this case differ from Case 1?
> What would your concerns be in working with the man in Case 2?

Case 1: Christine got pregnant in her first year of college. She had the baby and six months later she and the child's father married. Though she left school briefly, she registered at a local college and managed to re-establish her dream of a college education. She is more mature now than she would ever have been had she followed the path first laid down for her. She's certain of that. The marriage is strong, her child a blessing, and her bachelor's degree is within sight. The question now is what to do next. The career counselor at the school thinks she should consider law school. Friends tell her that she would make an excellent counselor. Christine thinks of having more children, too, but is uncertain how many she should have. Fortunately, there is enough money to realistically consider these options and others. She knows that she has to make some important decisions, so she comes to you for help.

Case 2: Ray, 41 years old, is a middle manager in a manufacturing company located in a large city. He goes to see a counselor with a somewhat complex story. He is bored with his job; his marriage is lifeless; he has poor rapport with his two teenage children, one of whom is having trouble with drugs; he is drinking heavily; he doesn't think much of himself; he has begun to steal things, small things, not because he needs them but because he gets a kick out of it. He tells his story in a rather disjointed way, skipping around from one problem area to another. He is a talented, personable, engaging man who seems to be adrift in life. He does not show any symptoms of severe psychiatric illness. He does experience a great deal of uneasiness in talking about himself. This is his first visit to a helper.

EXERCISE 10.6: CHOOSING ISSUES THAT MAKE A DIFFERENCE

As you just read with Christine and Ray, the stories clients tell are often quite complex, so they may need your help in deciding which issues to work on first and which merit substantial attention. In this exercise you are asked to review the examples of Christine and Ray.

1. Briefly list any concerns that were noted for each of these clients.

Christine: _____

_____

_____

_____

_____

Ray: _____

_____

_____

_____

_____

_____

2. Next, do some screening. Put a line through any of these issues that you believe probably do not warrant counseling or should be addressed in another manner.
3. Review the remaining items on each list in the light of the following "leverage" criteria:

- If there is a crisis, first help the client manage the crisis.
- Begin with the problem that seems to be causing pain for the client.
- Begin with issues the client sees as important and is motivated to work on.
- Begin with some manageable sub-problem of a larger problem situation.

117

- Begin with a problem that, if handled, will lead to some kind of general improvement in the client's condition.
- Focus on a problem for which the benefits will outweigh the costs.

4. Rank order the items listed for each client. Then share the rankings with a learning partner. Explain the "leverage" reasons behind your rankings. Explain your choices and rankings in terms of the criteria outlined above or any further criteria not listed there. What is the value, the "bang for the buck," of each?

PULLING STAGE I TOGETHER

The following exercise asks you to pull together what you have learned about Stage I of the helping process and apply it to yourself.

EXERCISE 10.7: COUNSELING YOURSELF: AN EXERCISE IN STAGE I

At this point, you have developed an overview of the problem-management framework and, through reading and doing the exercises in this workbook, developed an understanding and behavioral "feel" for Stage I. In this exercise you are asked to carry on a dialogue with yourself in writing. Choose a problematic area of your life or some unexploited opportunity—something that is relevant to your success as a helper. First use empathic highlights, probes, and challenges to help yourself tell your story. Work at clarifying it in terms of specific experiences, behaviors, and feelings. Explore your own points of view. Clarify your decisions. Take a closer look at intended courses of action related to the issue you choose. Both probe and challenge yourself with respect to the "little" actions you can take to manage this problem or opportunity.

Example: This example comes from the experience of Cora, a woman in a master's degree program in counseling psychology. Here is some of her dialogue with herself.

Her initial story. "To be frank, I have a number of misgivings about becoming a counselor. A number of things are turning me off. For instance, one of my instructors this past semester was an arrogant guy. I kept saying to myself, 'Is this what these psychology programs produce? Could this guy really help anyone?' I also find the program much too theoretical. In a Theories of Counseling and Psychotherapy course we never did anything, not even discuss the practical implications of these theories. And so they remained just that—theories. I'm very disappointed. I'm about to go into my second year, but I have serious reservations. From what others tell me, the program gets a bit more practical, but not enough. There's a practicum experience at the end of the program, but I want more hands-on work now. So I've started working at a halfway house for people discharged from mental hospitals. But that's not working out the way I expected either. There's something about this whole helping business that is making me think twice about myself and about the profession."

SELF-COUNSELOR: All of this adds up to the fact that the helping profession, at least from your experience, is not what it's cracked up to be. The program and some of the instructors in it have left you quite disappointed. Of all these issues, which one or ones hits you the hardest?
SELF-CLIENT: Hmm. It's hard to say, but I think the halfway house bothers me most. Because that's not theoretical stuff. That's real stuff out there.
SELF-COUNSELOR: That's a place where real helping should be taking place. But you've got misgivings about what's going on there.
SELF-CLIENT: Yes, two sets of misgivings. One set about me and one about the place.
SELF-COUNSELOR: Tell me more about one set or the other.

SELF-CLIENT: I feel I have to explore both, but I'll start with myself. I felt so ill-prepared for what I encountered. What's in the lectures and books seems so distant from the realities of the halfway house. For instance, the other day one of the residents there began yelling at me when we were passing in the hallway. She hit me a few times and then ran off screaming that I was trying to get her in some way. I didn't know what to do. I felt so incompetent. And I felt guilty.

SELF-COUNSELOR: That sounds pretty upsetting. You just weren't prepared for it. I'm wondering whether the more practical part of the counseling program you're going into would better prepare you for that kind of reality.

SELF-CLIENT: It could be. I may be doing myself in by jumping ahead of myself.

SELF-COUNSELOR: But you still have reservations about the effectiveness of the halfway house.

SELF-CLIENT: I wasn't ready for what I found there. I've been there a couple of months. No one has really helped me learn the ropes. I don't have an official supervisor. I just see all sorts of people with problems and help when I can.

SELF-COUNSELOR: You just don't feel prepared and they don't do much to help you. So you feel inadequate. You also seem to be basing your judgments about the adequacy of helper-training programs and helping facilities in general, on your experience in this training program, and on the halfway house.

SELF-CLIENT: That's a good point. I'm making the assumption that both should be high-quality places. As far as I can tell, they're not. I guess I have to work on myself first. But that's why I went to the halfway house in the first place. I'm an independent person, but I'm too much on my own there. In a sense, I'm trusted, but, since I don't get much supervision, I have to go on my own instincts and I'm not sure they're always right.

SELF-COUNSELOR: There's some comfort in being trusted, but without supervision you still have a what-am-I-doing-here feeling.

SELF-CLIENT: Right. There are many times when I ask myself just that, "What are you doing here?" I provide day-to-day services for a lot of people. I listen to them. I take them places, like to the doctor. I get them to participate in conversations or games and things like that. But it seems that I'm always just meeting the needs of the moment. I'm not sure what the long-range goals of the place are and if anyone, including me, is contributing to them in any way.

SELF-COUNSELOR: You seem to have started with a rather difficult population. You get some satisfaction in providing the services you do, but you don't feel equipped to add real value in the halfway house. You may even wonder what this value might look like. Anyway, the lack of overall purpose or direction for yourself and the institution is frustrating. I'm not sure whether you've asked yourself what you might do about all of this, either at the halfway house or in the counseling program.

SELF-CLIENT: I'm letting myself get frustrated, irritated, and depressed. I'm down on myself and down on the people who run the house. It's a day-to-day operation that sometimes seems to be a fly-by-night venture. See! There I go. You're right. I'm not doing anything to handle my frustrations. I'm just blaming everyone else. And I'm doing little to try to better myself. I'm just beginning to put it into some kind of context.

SELF-COUNSELOR: So this is really the first time you've stopped to take a critical look at yourself as a potential helper and the settings in which helping takes place. And what you see is depressing.

SELF-CLIENT: Absolutely.

SELF-COUNSELOR: I wonder how fair you're being to yourself, to the profession, and even to the halfway house.

SELF-CLIENT (Pause): Well, that's a point. I'm speaking — and making judgments — out of a great deal of frustration. I don't want to go off half-cocked. But I could share my concerns about the psychology program with one of the instructors. She teaches the second-year trainees. She gave a very practical talk. I could also see whether my concerns are shared by my classmates. I could also talk to the second-year students to get a feeling for how practical next year might be.

SELF-COUNSELOR: All in all, you can give yourself a chance to get a more balanced perspective.

SELF-CLIENT: Right. I need to do something instead of just brooding and complaining. But there's still the halfway house. I don't want to come across as the wet-behind-the-ears critic.

SELF-COUNSELOR: I'm not sure whether you're assuming that halfway house you're working in should be a state-of-the-art facility?

SELF-CLIENT: Touché! . . . . Wow, I am basing a lot of my feelings about the profession on that place.

SELF-COUNSELOR: Who at the house might you trust to help you get a better perspective?

SELF-CLIENT: Well, hmm . . . There is a consultant who shows up once in a while. He runs staff meetings. And he does it in a very practical way. Maybe I can get hold of him and get a better picture.

SELF-COUNSELOR: So, overall?

SELF-CLIENT: I've got some work to do before I rush to judgment. I like the fact that I want the people and the institutions in the profession to be competent. Deep down I think that I'd make a good helper. I say to myself, "You're all right; you're trying to do what is right." Also, I need to challenge my idealism. I spend too much time grieving over what is happening — or not happening — at school and at the halfway house. I need a more mature outlook and I need to figure out how to turn minuses into pluses, including my own.

1. Review this trainee's responses to herself with a learning partner. What kinds of responses did she use? How would you evaluate their quality? What progress did she make? Describe the movement she made during the session. What responses would you have changed?

2. Next choose a problematic area that is important to you—ideally, one involving both problems and unused opportunities—and then, on separate sheets of paper, write out a helping dialogue with yourself like the one above.

3. Exchange dialogues with your learning partner and critique what you have written in terms of the process and skills of Stage I outlined and illustrated in Chapters 3 – 7.

Chapter 11

STAGE II: DESIGNING THE FUTURE
TASK II-A: POSSIBILITIES FOR A BETTER FUTURE

Problems can make clients feel hemmed in and closed off. To a greater or lesser extent they have no future, or the future they have looks troubled. But, as Gelatt (1989) noted, "The future does not exist and cannot be predicted. It must be imagined and invented." (p. 255) The interrelated tasks of Stage II outline three ways in which helpers can partner with their clients with a view to exploring and developing this better future.

Task A—Possibilities. "What possibilities do I have for a better future?" "What would my life look like if it looked better?" In helping clients move from problems to solutions, counselors help them develop a sense of hope.

Task B—Choices. "What do I really want and need? What solutions are best for me?" Here counselors help clients craft a viable change agenda from among the possibilities. Helping them shape this agenda is the central task of helping.

Task C—Commitment. "What am I willing to pay for what I want?" Help clients discover incentives for commitment to their change agenda. It is a further look at the economics of personal change discussed in Task C of Stage I.

TASK II-A:
HELP CLIENTS DISCOVER POSSIBILITIES FOR A BETTER FUTURE
"What Would a Better Life Look Like?"

Effective helping requires imagination. In this task you help clients develop a vision of a better future. Once clients understand the nature of the problem situation or identify a key unused opportunity, they need to ask themselves, "What do I want? What would my situation look like if it were better, at least a little bit better?" Read Chapter 11 before doing these exercises.

EXERCISE 11.1: THERAPY—SCIENCE, ENGINEERING, OR ART?

There are what some call the STEM (science, technology, engineering, mathematics) professions. Designing, building, and landing the Mars Rover involved all of these. Therapy is often described as a combination of art and science. It might be better to say that the helping professions involve a kind of art, a kind of engineering, and a kind of science. Given what you know about the elements of successful therapy so far and the use you have made of these elements, what is your understanding of how a kind of art, a kind of engineering, and a kind of science intermingle in what we call therapy?

1. Answer the following questions in the order that makes most sense to you. If you choose a particular order, muse on why you are doing so.

List some ways that therapy is an art.

_____

_____

_____

_____

List some way in which therapy is a kind of engineering.

_____

_____

_____

_____

List some ways in which therapy involves one kind of science (social science).

_____

_____

_____

_____

2. Discuss your answers to the following questions with a learning partner: Why did you choose the order you took? How do these three dimensions of therapy overlap and intermingle? How does each element add value to the other two?

EXERCISE 11.2: PROBLEMS AND UNUSED OPPORTUNITIES IN THE SOCIAL SETTINGS OF LIFE

This is another exercise that will help you review areas in which clients have problems and also help you identify your own strengths and weaknesses. Individuals belong to and participate in a number of different social settings in life: family, circle of friends, clubs, church groups, school groups, work groups, and the like. People are also affected by what goes on in their neighborhoods and the cities and towns in which they live. Larger systems, such as state and national governments, have their ways of entering people's lives.

1. Chart the social settings of your life as in the example below. The person in the example is Mitch, 45, a principal of an inner-city high school in a large city. He is married and has two teenage sons. Neither son attends the high school of which he is principal. He is seeing a counselor because of exhaustion and bouts of hostility and depression. He has had a complete physical check-up and there is no evidence of any medical problem.

2. Choose two or three social settings that are currently important in your life. These are settings in which you are experiencing problems or have unused opportunities.

3. Review issues, demands, conflicts, concerns. Now take each key social setting and write down issues or concerns in that setting. For instance, some of things Mitch writes are:

School
- Some faculty members want a personal relationship with me and I have neither the time nor the desire.
- Some faculty members have retired on the job. I don't know what to do with them.
- Some of the white faculty members are suspicious of me and distant just because I'm black.
- One faculty member wrote the district superintendent and said that I was undermining her reputation with other faculty members. This is not true.

122

- The students, both individually and through their organizations, keep asking me to be more liberal while their parents are asking me to tighten things up.

Family
- My wife says that I'm letting school consume me; she complains constantly because I don't spend enough time at home. Even though she wants me to spend more time at home, she criticizes me for not spending more time with my parents.
- My kids seem to withdraw from me because I'm a double authority figure, a father and a principal.

Parents
- My mother is infirm; my retired father calls me and tells me what a hard time he's having getting used to retirement.
- My mother tells me not to be spending time with her when I have so much to do and then she complains to my wife and my father when I don't show up.

School District
- I would like to become the district superintendent. I think I could do a lot of good.

Friends
- My friends say that I spend so much time at work involving myself in crisis management that I have no time left for them; they tell me I'm doing myself in.

4. Review possibilities for a better future. Choose two concerns arising from two different social settings of your life. Spell out some of the possibilities for a better future in this area. What would this problem or unused opportunity look like if it were managed better or solved? What are some of the things that would be in place that are not now in place? Use the following probes to help yourself brainstorm possibilities.

- Here's what I need . . . .
- Here's what I want . . . .
- Here are some items on my wish list . . . .
- When I'm finished I will have . . . .
- There will be . . . .
- Will have in place . . . .
- I will consistently be . . . .
- There will be more of . . . .
- There will be less of . . . .

For instance, Mitch, in reviewing the conflict between his work and his friends, comes up with these possibilities: more time with his friends, greater flexibility in managing his calendar at work, better integration of his friendships with his home life, a more clear-cut division between his work setting and the other social settings of his life, more time for himself, a clearer understanding of his career aspirations and the costs associated with them, and better delegation on his part to the members of the school administrative team. These are all possibilities for a better future. Now do the same for yourself. Use a separate piece of paper to map out the social settings of your life (as Mitch did).

First social setting.

_____

_____

Key issues, concerns, demands, conflicts, and unused opportunities in this social setting.

_____

_____

_____

_____

_____

Possibilities for a better future in this social setting.

_____

_____

_____

_____

_____

Second social setting.

_____

_____

Key issues, concerns, demands, conflicts and unused opportunities in this social setting.

_____

_____

_____

_____

Possibilities for a better future in this area of concern.

_____

_____

_____

_____

_____

5. Review your findings with a learning partner.

EXERCISE 11.3: BRAINSTORMING POSSIBILITIES FOR A BETTER FUTURE—CASES

This exercise focuses on a number of cases, many of which you have seen before. Now you are asked to put yourself in each person's shoes and brainstorm possibilities for a better future. What would things look like if they looked better? If you were this person, what are some of the things you would want instead of what you've got?

1. Read the case. Put yourself in this person's shoes. Make his or her problem situation your own.
2. Brainstorm a number of possibilities for a better future. What would you want if you were this person?

Case 1. Tim was a bright, personable young man. During college he was hospitalized after taking a drug overdose during a bout of depression. He spent six months as an in-patient. He was assigned to "milieu therapy," an amorphous mixture of work and recreation designed more to keep patients busy than to help them grapple with their problems and engage in constructive change. He was given drugs for his depression, seen occasionally by a psychiatrist, and assigned to a therapy group that proved to be quite aimless. After leaving the hospital, his confidence shattered, he left college and got involved with a variety of low-paying, part-time jobs. He finally finished college by going to night school, but he avoided full-time jobs for fear of being asked about his past. Buried inside him was the thought, "I have this terrible secret that I have to keep from everyone." A friend talked him into taking a college-sponsored communication-skills course one summer. The psychologist running the program, noting Tim's rather substantial natural talents together with his self-effacing ways, remarked to him one day, "I wonder what kind of ambitions you have." In an instant Tim realized that he had buried all thoughts of ambition. After all, he didn't "deserve" to be ambitious. Tim, instinctively trusting the program director, divulged the "terrible secret" about his hospitalization for the first time.

Jot down a range of possibilities for a better future.

_____

_____

_____

_____

_____

Case 2. A nun, 44 years old, a member of a counselor training group, has been talking about her dissatisfaction with her present job. Although a nurse, she is presently teaching in a primary school because, she says, of the "urgent needs" of that school. When pressed, she refers briefly to a history of job dissatisfaction. In the group she has shown herself to be an active, intelligent, and caring woman who tends to speak and act in self-effacing ways. She mentions how obedience has been stressed throughout her years in the religious order. She does mention, however, that things have been "letting up a bit" in recent years. The younger sisters don't seem to be as preoccupied with obedience as she is. She says:

"The reason I'm talking about my job is that I don't want to become a counselor and then discover it's another job I'm dissatisfied with. It would be unfair to the people I'd be working with and unfair to my religious order, which is paying for my education. Of course, I have no iron-clad assurance that I'll be put in a job that will enable me to use my counselor training."

A range of possibilities for a better future.

_____

_____

_____

_____

Case 3. Marcus, 47 years old, is a successful businessman whose life is in fairly good order. However, Yves, his younger brother, is struggling financially. His credit-card debt is enormous. For Marcus the problem is how to extend a helping hand to his younger brother without robbing him of his self-responsibility. He explains his dilemma to a colleague at work, "Yves is very sensitive to this older brother-younger brother stuff. Anyway, he has it in his head that I see him as incompetent and any help I offer is seen through that filter. I suppose that I'll always be the successful big brother and he will always be the inept little brother. It's not that way really but.... What I can't do is let our past history force me to stand off to the side with my hands in my pockets and do nothing when I know I could be of some help. I'm not sure what kind of help would make sense."

A range of possibilities for a better future.

_____

_____

_____

_____

Case 4. This man, now 64 years old, retired early from work when he was 62. He and his wife wanted to take full advantage of the "golden" years. But his wife died a year after he retired. At the urging of friends he has finally come to a counselor. He has been exploring some of the problems his retirement has created for him. His two married sons live with their families in other cities. In the counseling sessions he has been dealing somewhat repetitiously with the theme of loss. He says: "I seldom see the kids. I enjoy them and their families a lot when they do come. I get along real well with their wives. But now that my wife is gone. . . (pause). . . and since I've stopped working . . . (pause) . . . I seem to just ramble around the house aimlessly, which is not like me at all. I suppose I should get rid of the house, but it's filled with a lot of memories—bittersweet memories now. There were a lot of good years here."

A range of possibilities for a better future.

_____

_____

_____

_____

EXERCISE 11.4: HELPING SOMEONE DEVELOP POSSIBILITIES FOR A BETTER FUTURE

In this exercise, you are asked to help one of the other members of your group develop possibilities for a better future.

1. Divide up into groups of three for this exercise.
2. Assume, sequentially, the roles of client, helper, and observer.
3. In the role of client, provide a summary of one of the problem situations or undeveloped opportunities you focused on in any of the previous exercises. Or, if you prefer, choose a new issue.
4. In the role of counselor, listen to your partner summarize his or her problem situation or undeveloped opportunity. Use empathy and probes to get a full statement of the issue.
5. Finally, help the other develop possibilities for a better future. Use empathy, probes, summaries, and invitations to self-challenge to help the other expand the list.

Example: Michael, a junior in college majoring in business studies, has given the following summary of the problem situation: "My uncle runs a small business. He's offered me a kind of internship in the family business. While such an opportunity fits perfectly with my career plans, I have done nothing to develop it. Right now, it's only an interesting idea. But it still seems too good an opportunity to miss." Trish, his helper, uses all the communication skills learned up to this point to help him develop possibilities for a productive internship. Some of the dialogue goes like this:

TRISH: So you haven't taken the time yet to spell out what the internship could look like.
MICHAEL: No. Generally, I see the internship as something that would bring to life the stuff I'm getting out of business books right now.
TRISH: So the internship would give you a chance for some hands-on experience with business realities that are just concepts now. What could the internship look like?
MICHAEL: Well, I don't know what's on my uncle's mind. Though he's not going to push me into anything I don't want.
TRISH: Then it seems to make sense for you to have some ideas in mind before you talk with him about it. What would _you_ like the internship to look like? What do you want?
MICHAEL: Let's see. I'd be putting in 10 to 15 hours a week at my uncle's business. Actually, that would make sense since I'm more or less overbalanced right now on social activities.
TRISH: What would you be doing during those hours?
MICHAEL: Well, I don't like the finance part of my program. So one thing I could do is become familiar with the finance part of his business—where the money comes from, what kind of debt he carries, cash flow—all those things that are still too theoretical for me in the courses I'm taking.
TRISH: You'd see finance in action. It might even seem more interesting to you then. What else do you picture yourself doing?

MICHAEL: I like to find out what management and supervision actually looks like inside a company. I get a confused picture of both of these from what I'm reading.

TRISH: So it's one thing to read management books, but another to see how it actually works. What might you do as a manager or supervisor?

MICHAEL: I'm not sure he'd let me run anything important. But maybe I could run a project or two. And the project might involve working with others—you know, like a small team. I think I'd like to see how teamwork can affect the business. I guess what I'm saying is that my uncle's business could be a lab for me. I'd be contributing, but also I'd be learning a lot.

TRISH: So project work and teamwork could be important parts of the lab. But it also sounds like you want to be a contributor in all this.

MICHAEL. Yeah. I'd like to learn, but I'd like to make a difference.

TRISH. What kind of difference?

The dialogue goes on in that vein. Michael, with the help of Trish, develops a lot of possibilities for the internship.

1. With your partner, critique this dialogue. What did Trish do well? What might have been done better?
2. Then move on to your own dialogue. The client starts with a summary of a problem situation or unused opportunity. Video the session.
3. In the role of counselor, help your client expand on his or her summary of the problem situation so that it is clear and has substance.
4. Next help your client brainstorm some possibilities for a better future. What would the problem situation look like down the road if it was being managed well? Spend about ten minutes.
5. At the end of the session, the client gives feedback in two areas. First, what kind of progress was made? Second, how well did the helper do his or her job? Finally, the observer gives his overall evaluation of the session.
6. Repeat the process until each person has played each role.

EXERCISE 11.5: REVIEWING THE "SHADOW SIDE" OF YOUR DECISION MAKING STYLE

In the next three chapters you are going to be reviewing the elements that go into effective goal setting, planning, and implementation of plans. Decision making plays a large role in these processes. As mentioned in Chapter 1, helping clients make decisions about making changes is one of the key ingredients of successful therapy. Decision making is at the heart of therapy. If clients understand their decision-making style, they have a better chance of making life-enhancing decisions. For example, an organizational manager who makes decisions based only on facts (i.e., the bottom line) may end up with unhappy employees, high turnover, and poor productivity. On the other hand, if a manager makes decisions based only on trying to make her employees happy, the company might go out of business. There is no one right way to make a good decision.

As mentioned in Chapter 1, there are many obstacles both within the environment and within our heads to making effective life-enhancing decisions. In this exercise you are asked to become more familiar with these obstacles. A number of books detailing the "shadow side" of decision making were cited in Chapter 1.

1. Find and read some articles or even a book on the nonrational factors in decision making.

2. Reflect on your own experience and list a few of these factors that might affect the way you make decisions.

_____

_____

_____

_____

_____

3. Think of someone you know who, in your estimation, tends to make poor decisions. Jot down a few reasons for his or her poor decisions.

_____

_____

_____

_____

_____

4. Discuss what you learned about your and other people's decision-making style with a learning partner. How can you make better decisions? How can you help others make better decisions?

EXERCISE 11.6: HELPING CLIENTS EXPLORE THE WAY THEY MAKE DECISIONS

If you are to help clients make better decisions, it is important to understand how clients go about making decisions or what makes them hesitate to make life-enhancing decisions.

1. Form groups of three: client, helper, observer.
2. The client describes a situation of reasonable substance that involves a decision of some importance. Clients may be: (a) uncertain about whether they truly want to make a change in their lives, (b) certain that they want to make a change in their lives, but are unsure how to do it, or (c) certain both that they want to make a change in their lives and how to make a change.
3. The client summarizes the situation that involves making a decision.
4. For about 10 minutes, the helper uses his or her skills to help the client explore the decision (or decisions) involved in the problem situation and/or unused opportunity. Video the session.
5. After the session, the three participants debrief the interaction with the help of the video. The client takes the lead in providing feedback. The observer chimes in, and the helper provides feedback to himself or herself. To what degree was there some positive outcome? What did the client learn about his or her decision-making style? How effective was the helper in "nudging" the client to some kind of life-enhancing decision? What could have been done better?
6. Change roles and repeat the exercise.

Chapter 12

STAGE II
TASK II-B: GOALS, OUTCOMES, IMPACT
TASK II-C: COMMITMENT

TASK II-B:
HELP CLIENTS MOVE FROM POSSIBILITIES TO CHOICES
"What Solutions Are Best for Me?"

Once clients have brainstormed possibilities for a better future, they need to make some choices. Answers to the questions, "What do you want" and "What do you need?" are possible goals. Answers to the question, "What do you really need and want?" are the actual goals that constitute the change agenda. It is as if the client were to say, "Here is what I want in place of what I have right now." Goals are a critical part of an agenda for constructive change. For instance, Michael, the college student mentioned in Chapter 11, after brainstorming a number of possibilities for structuring his internship in his uncle's company, chooses four of the possibilities and makes these his agenda. He shares them with his uncle and, after some negotiation, comes up with a revised package they can both live with. Review Chapter 12, Task II-B in the text before doing the exercises below.

EXERCISE 12.1: TURNING POSSIBILITIES INTO GOALS—A CASE

In this exercise you are asked to do what Michael had to do—choose goals from among the possibilities. Possibilities should be chosen because they will best help you manage your problem situation or develop some opportunity. First, read the following case.

The Case. Vanessa, a 46-year-old Latina woman, has been divorced for about a year. She has done little to restructure her life and is still in the doldrums. At the urging of a friend, she sees a counselor. With the counselor's help, she brainstorms a range of possibilities for a better future around the theme of "my new life as a single person." She is currently a salesperson in the women's apparel department of a moderately upscale store. She lives in the house that was part of the divorce settlement. She has no children. When she finally decided that she wanted children, it was too late. There was some discussion with her ex-husband about adopting a child, but it didn't get very far. The marriage was already disintegrating. Her visits to the counselor have reawakened a desire to take charge of her life and not just let it happen. She let her marriage happen and it fell apart. She is not filled with anger at her former husband. If anything, she's a bit too down on herself. Her grieving is filled with self-recrimination.

     The helper asks her, "What do you want now that the divorce is final? What would you like your post-divorce life to look like? What would you want to see in place?" Vanessa brainstorms the following possibilities:

- A job in some area of the fashion industry.
- A small condo that will not need much maintenance on my part instead of the house.
- The elimination of poor-me attitudes as part of a much more creative outlook on self and life.
- The elimination of waiting around for things to happen.
- The development of a social life. For the time being, a range of friends rather than potential husbands. A couple of good women friends.
- Getting into physical shape.

130

- A hobby or avocation that I could get lost in. Something with substance.
- Some sort of volunteer work. With children, if possible.
- Some religion-related activities, not necessarily established-church related. Something that deals with the "bigger" questions of life.
- An end to all the self-recrimination over the divorce.
- Resetting my relationship with my mother (who strongly disapproved of the divorce).
- Getting over a deep-seated fear that my life is going to be bland, if not actually bleak.
- Possibly some involvement with politics.

1. Read the list from Vanessa's point of view (even though you don't really know her).
2. Because Vanessa cannot possibly do all of these at once, she has to make some choices. Put yourself in her place. Which items would you include in your agenda if you were Vanessa? In what way would the agenda items, if accomplished, help manage the overall problem situation and develop opportunities?
3. Choose three and give your reasons for including each.
4. Share your package together with the reasons for each item in it with a learning partner.
5. Discuss the differences in the items chosen and the reasons for the choices. Note that there is no one right package.

My first choice.

_____

_____

My reason for the choice.

_____

_____

My second choice.

_____

_____

My reason for the choice.

_____

_____

_____

My third choice.

_____

_____

My reason for the choice.

_____

_____

EXERCISE 12.2: TURNING PERSONAL POSSIBILITIES INTO PERSONAL GOALS

In this exercise you are asked to review **EXERCISE 11.2: PROBLEMS AND OPPORTUNITIES IN THE SOCIAL SETTINGS OF LIFE** in which you brainstormed a range of possibilities for a better future for yourself.

1. Pick two of the three social settings you explored.
2. In each, after reviewing the possibilities that you brainstormed, come up with a goal and your reason for it.
3. Use the criteria outlined in Chapter 12 in order to "fashion" or "design" the goals.
After completing the exercise, share and critique your goals with a learning partner.

1. First social setting.

_____

_____

Goal for this setting.

_____

_____

Reason for the goal.

_____

_____

2. Second social-setting.

_____

_____

Goal for this setting.

_____

_____

Reason for the goal.

_____

_____

EXERCISE 12.3: HELPING CLIENTS TURN POSSIBILITIES INTO GOALS

In this exercise you are asked to review **EXERCISE 11.3: BRAINSTORMING POSSIBILITIES FOR A BETTER FUTURE—CASES** in which you brainstormed a range of possibilities for a better future for three different clients.

1. Pick two of the three cases in that exercise.
2. In each, turn the possibilities that you brainstormed into a workable goal or set of goals.
3. Use the criteria outlined in Chapter 12 to "fashion" or "design" the goals.
4. After completing the exercise, share and critique your goals with a learning partner.

1. First case.

_____

_____

Possibilities turned into a goal.

_____

_____

_____

Reason for the goal

_____

_____

_____

2. Second case.

_____

_____

Possibilities turned into a goal.

_____

_____

_____

Reason for the goal.

_____

_____

_____

EXERCISE 12.4: SHAPING GOALS—FROM BROAD TO SPECIFIC

Many clients set goals that are too vague to be accomplished. "I'm going to clean up my act" is nothing more than a good intention. It is not yet a goal. Part of shaping, then, is making goals specific enough to drive action. This exercise involves moving from vagueness to concreteness.

1. First, evaluate the goal Tom and Carol (in the example below) have set for themselves in terms of its specificity. If you don't think it is specific enough, shape it—that is, make it more specific.
2. Then, in the cases that follow, get inside the client's mind and try to determine what he or she might need or want.
3. Then, move from a vaguely stated good intention to a broad aim and then to a specific goal.
4. Finally, learning partners should share the goals they have written and provide feedback for each other. When necessary, goals should be reformulated.

Example: Tom, 42, and his wife, Carol, 39, have been talking to a counselor about how poorly they relate to each other. They have explored their own behavior in concrete ways, have developed a variety of new perspectives on themselves as both individuals and as a couple, and now want to do something about what they have learned. In broad terms, they have agreed to stop blaming each other for their problems and take mutual responsibility for creating a better relationship. What follows is their first shot at moving from a vague to a more specific goal in the area of communication:

Good Intention: "We've got to do something about the way we communicate with each other. It's just not healthy."
General Aim: "We are constantly at each other over inconsequential issues and then it escalates. We'd like to do something about the way we bicker."
Specific Goal(s): "We want to call a moratorium on what has become almost childish bickering. We want to stop second-guessing, picking on, correcting, one-upping, putting down, questioning, and being hurtful to each other. But we don't want to leave a vacuum. We need something positive to take its place. For instance, when we kid around, each of us should make himself or herself, not the other, the butt of any joke. When we do disagree about something important, we should avoid overly personal heated arguments and instead engage in mutual problem solving based on the skilled helping process we are using in counseling."

First, critique the specific goals in the above example and then work on the cases below.

1. Sherry, a 42-year-old single White woman, just had her annual physical and was told that she needs to lose weight and improve her health. She was prescribed medication for both high blood pressure and cholesterol. She is a long time smoker (a pack a day) and self-confessed "chocaholic." Sherry readily acknowledges that she needs to change the way she lives and to take better care of herself, but says "Trying to raise two teenagers and work full-time makes eating healthy and exercising regularly really hard."

Statement of good intention.

_____

_____

Broad aim.

_____

_____

Specific goal(s).

_____

_____

2. Troy, 30, has been discussing the stress he has been experiencing during this transitional year of his life. Part of the stress relates to his job. He has been working as an accountant with a large firm for the past five years. He makes a decent salary, but he is more and more dissatisfied with the kind of work he is doing. He finds accounting predictable and boring. He doesn't feel that there's much chance for advancement in this company. Many of his associates are much more ambitious and much more inventive than he is.

Statement of good intention.

_____

_____

Broad aim.

_____

_____

Specific goal.

_____

_____

3. Bob, a 65-year-old engineer, has been offered an early retirement package as part of a company restructuring strategy to save money. Bob has always enjoyed his work but also realizes that he needs to start thinking about when he wants to retire and how we would spend his time. Thinking about it is both exciting and scary for him. His identity has been one of a successful engineer, and he feels as if he wants to retire on his terms and not the company's, but he is also intrigued by the possibilities of having time to learn and try new things. He has thought about wanting to travel, teaching math courses at the local college, learning how to play the guitar, and simply having more time to spend with his children and grandchildren. So many possibilities!

Statement of good intention.

_____

_____

Broad aim.

_____

_____

_____

Specific goal.

_____

_____

4. Len, married with three teenage children, lost all the family's savings in a gambling spree. Under a lot of pressure from both his family and his boss, he started attending Gamblers Anonymous meetings. He seemed to recover—that is, he stopped betting on horses and ball games. A couple of years went by and Len stopped going to the GA meetings because he "no longer needed them." He even got a better job and was recovering financially quite well. But his wife began to notice that he was on the phone a great deal with his broker. She confronted him and he reluctantly agreed to a session with one of the friends he made at GA. He says, "She's worried that I'm gambling again. You know, it's really just the opposite. When I was gambling, I was financially irresponsible. I lost our future on horses and ball games. But now I'm taking a very active part in creating our financial future. Every financial planner will tell you that investing in the market is central to sound financial planning. I'm a doer. I'm taking a very active role."

Statement of good intention.

_____

_____

Broad aim.

_____

_____

Specific goal.

_____

_____

5. Jaime, a 32-year old married woman, has two small children. Her husband has left her and she has no idea where he is. She has no relatives in the city and only a few acquaintances. She is talking to a counselor in a local community center about her plight. Since her husband was the breadwinner, she now has no income and no savings on which to draw.

Statement of good intention.

_____

_____

Broad aim.

_____

_____

Specific goal.

_____

_____

EXERCISE 12.5: SHAPING GOALS—MAKING SURE THAT THEY ARE WORKABLE

Accomplishing goals is a lot of work. If the goals chosen are themselves flawed, then the job becomes almost impossible. For instance, if Dylan chooses a career for which he does not have the talent, he is doing himself no favor. Hard work won't make up for the talent deficit. In order to be workable, goals generally need to be:

- stated as outcomes,
- specific enough to drive action,
- substantial enough to make a difference,
- characterized by the right mixture of risk and prudence,
- realistic,
- sustainable,
- flexible,
- congruent with the client's values,
- set in a reasonable time frame.

These characteristics can be seen as tools that help you shape both your own and clients' goals.

1. With a learning partner return to the four goals that each of you set in exercises 12.2 and 12.3. Use the above characteristics to review them once more.
2. What changes might you make in each of these goals to make them conform to the above characteristics?

EXERCISE 12.6: HELPING LEARNING PARTNERS SET WORKABLE GOALS

In this exercise you are asked to act as a helper to a learning partner. This exercise is done verbally.

1. The total training group is to be divided up into smaller groups of three.
2. There are three roles: client, helper, and observer. Decide the order in which you will play each role. It would be helpful to video the session.
3. The client summarizes some problem situation (real or imagined) and then declares his or her intent to do something about the problem or some part of it.
4. The group member in helper role, using empathic highlights, probing, and invitations to self-challenge, helps the client move from this statement of intent to a broad aim and then to a specific problem-managing or opportunity-developing goal that has the characteristics listed above.
5. When the helper feels that he or she has fulfilled this task, the session is ended. Both the observer and client then give specific feedback to the helper on at least three things that they liked and one or more things that could be improved.
6. Repeat the process until each person has played each role.

Example: Emilia, a junior beginning her third year of college, is dissatisfied with the way she goes about learning. She decides to use her imagination to invent a more creative approach to study. She brainstorms possibilities for a better study future, that is, goals that would constitute her new learning style. She says to herself: "In my role as student or learner, what do I want? Let me brainstorm the possibilities."

- I will stop studying for grades and start studying to learn. Paradoxically this might help my grades, but I will not be putting in extra effort just to raise a B to an A.
- I will be a better contributor in class, not in the sense that I will be trying to make a good impression on my teachers. I will do whatever I need to do to learn. This may mean placing more demands on teachers to clarify points, making more contributions, and involving myself in discussions with peers.
- I will be reading more broadly in the area of my major, psychology, not just the articles and books assigned but also in the areas of my interest. I will let my desire to know drive my learning.

She is particularly disappointed in the way she goes about writing the papers assigned in class. She believes that she wastes lots of time and ends up frustrated. And so she picks this topic for this exercise.

Declaration of intent: "I'm going to finally do something about the way I write papers for class."
Overall aim: "I'm going to put in place a systematic but flexible process for writing papers for class."

The task of the training group helper is to help Emilia develop and shape a problem-managing goal. Emilia begins by sharing her declaration of intent and overall aim. Here is some of the dialogue that follows:

JEREMY: What bothers you most about the way you have been doing your papers?
EMILIA: Everything piles up at the end and as a result the papers are rushed and practically never represent the kind of work I'm capable of.
JEREMY: So the unsystematic approach drives out quality. Let's see what a more systematic approach might look like. What are some of the elements of the process you want to put in place?
EMILIA: Well, I've thought about this a bit. For instance, once a paper is assigned, I will start a file on the topic and collect ideas, quotes, and data as I go along.
JEREMY: So you'll start early and have an organized filing system.
EMILIA: Yes. I'll start with a single folder and just throw in ideas or quotes from books or parts of lecture notes. Ideas from anywhere or everywhere. I'll sort them out later.
JEREMY: I wonder if the sorting process might become a bottleneck.
EMILIA: Hmm. You mean I'll end up with wads of stuff and wonder where to start. Well, there are two things I can do. I'll put only one item to a sheet of paper. One idea. One quote. You know. Then after two or three weeks I'll read through and separate them into different categories and organize them in folders.
JEREMY: The sub-category approach.
EMILIA: Right. Later on I can decide which topics are the most important ones. Then I can . . . .

Emilia and Jeremy go on in this vein until she has a clear idea of the process that she wants to put in place. When Emilia feels that she has a goal that will drive action, they stop and review and fine-tune the goal in terms of the goal characteristics outlined above. Prepare for your session with your helper by thinking of a statement of good intention and then by translating it into a broad goal. This is followed by a dialogue with a partner through which, with his or her help, you translate a broad intention into a workable goal.

Statement of good intention.

_____

_____

138

Broad aim.

_____

_____

Specific goal.

_____

_____

First, share your good intention and broad aim with your partner. Then have a goal-setting dialogue based on the criteria for effective goals. When finished, change roles.

EXERCISE 12.7: RELATING GOAL CHOICE TO ACTION

Once clients state what they want, they need to move into action in order to get what they want. At this point there are two ways of looking at the relationship of goals to action, one formal and one informal.

Formal Action. Stage III of the problem-management framework—brainstorming action strategies, choosing the best package, and turning them into a plan for accomplishing goals—is the formal approach to action.

Informal Action. Once clients get a fairly clear idea of what they want, there is no reason why they cannot move immediately into action, that is, do _something_ that will move them in the direction of their goals. These are the "little" actions that can precede the formal planning process. Indeed, these little actions can help clarify and fine-tune goals. This exercise is about these little actions.

1. State three personal goals that have emerged from your work in the training group.
2. For each goal list some "little actions" in which you might be able to engage in order to begin moving quickly in the direction of the goal.
3. Get feedback from a learning partner on both the goals and the actions.

Example. Review the case of Vanessa discussed above in Exercise 12.1. While she believes that it is essential for her to develop a better attitude about herself and life in general, she believes that it is not best to try to do this directly. Therefore, she chooses goals which will have a better attitude as a by-product.

One goal centers on the development of a social life. For the time being, she wants a range of friends rather than an intimate partner or potential spouse. She would especially like a couple of good women friends.

A second goal revolves around religion in some sense of that term. She would like to have religion-related activities, but not necessarily church-related, as part of her life. Something that deals with the "bigger" questions of life.

A third goal relates to physical well-being. The stress of the divorce has left her exhausted. She wants to build herself up physically and get into good physical shape.

Vanessa looks at the third goal and has this to say "There are some things I can do immediately without coming up with a formal physical fitness program. First of all exercise. I can begin by walking—to work, to the store, and so on. Second, I can easily cut down a lot on fast food and add some fresh fruit and vegetables to my diet. Let me try these two things and see where it leads." Now move on to your own personal goals.

139

First personal goal.

_____

_____

Actions you can take immediately.

_____

_____

_____

_____

Second personal goal.

_____

_____

Actions you can take immediately.

_____

_____

_____

_____

Third personal goal.

_____

_____

Actions you can take immediately.

_____

_____

_____

_____

TASK II-C:
HELP CLIENTS MAKE COMMITMENTS
"What Am I Willing to Pay for What I Want?"

Many of us choose goals that will help us manage problems and develop opportunities, but we do not explore the level of commitment that will be needed to pursue those goals successfully. Just because goals are tied nicely to the original problem situation and are initially espoused by us does not mean that we will follow through. Even goals which seem attractive from a cost/benefit point of view can fall by the wayside. The costs of accomplishing goals might not seem very high until it is time to pay up. Therefore, helping clients take a good look at commitment can raise the probability that they will actually pursue and accomplish these goals. Read the section on Task II-C in Chapter 12 before doing these exercises.

EXERCISE 12.8: MANAGING YOUR COMMITMENT TO YOUR GOALS

In this exercise you are asked to review the goals you have chosen to manage some problem situation or pursue some opportunity. The review should focus on commitment. It is not a question of challenging your good will. We all, at one time or another, make commitments that are not right for us.

1. Review the problem situations and unexploited opportunities you have been examining in this training program together with the goals you have established for yourself.
2. Choose two important goals you have decided to pursue.
3. Read the following questions and answer the ones you see as relevant to each goal in order to gauge your level of commitment:

- What is your state of readiness for change in this area at this time?
- To what degree are you choosing this goal freely?
- To what degree are you choosing this goal from among a number of possibilities?
- How appealing is this goal to you?
- Name any way in which your goal does not appeal to you.
- What's driving you to choose this goal?
- If your goal is in any way being imposed by others, what are you doing to make it your own? What incentives are there besides mere compliance?
- What difficulties are you experiencing in committing yourself to this goal?
- To what degree is it possible that your commitment is not a true commitment?
- What can you do to get rid of the disincentives and overcome the obstacles?
- What can you do to increase your commitment?
- In what ways can the goal be reformulated to make it more appealing?
- To what degree is the timing for pursuing this goal right or wrong?

Evaluation of your commitment to your first goal.

_____

_____

_____

_____

_____

Evaluation of your commitment to your second goal.

_____

_____

_____

_____

4. With a learning partner, review your principal learnings from answering the above questions about these two goals. Use empathic highlights, probes, and invitations to self-challenge to help each other explore levels of commitment.

5. Finally, to the degree necessary, reformulate both goals in terms of what you have learned from the dialogue.

Restated goal #1.

_____

_____

_____

_____

_____

Restated goal #2.

_____

_____

_____

_____

_____

EXERCISE 12.9: REVIEWING BENEFITS VERSUS COSTS IN CHOOSING GOALS

In most choices we make there are both benefits and costs. Commitment to a goal often depends on a favorable cost/benefit ratio. To what extent do the benefits outweigh the costs? The balance-sheet methodology outlined in Chapter 13 of *The Skilled Helper* can be useful in determining whether goals being chosen offer "value for money," as it were. Consider the following case.

Case. One January, Anna, a married Native American woman with two children (one a senior in college and one a sophomore) was told that she had an advanced case of cancer. She was also told that a rather rigorous series of chemotherapy treatments might prolong her life, but they would not save her. She desperately wanted to see her daughter graduate from college in June, so she opted for the treatments. Although she found them quite difficult, she buoyed herself up by the desire to be at the graduation. Although in a wheelchair, she was there for the graduation in June. When the doctor suggested that she could now face the inevitable with equanimity, she said: "But, doctor, in only two years my other son will be graduating."

This is a striking example of a woman's deciding that the costs, however high, were outweighed by the benefits. Obviously, this is not always the case. Benefits include incentives and rewards for whatever source, while costs include time and effort spent, resources used, psychological wear and tear, battling negative emotions, and the like. This exercise gives you the opportunity to explore your goals from a cost-benefit perspective. To what degree is it worth the effort? What's the payoff?

1. Divide up into pairs, with one partner acting as client, one as helper. Video the session.
2. Help your partner review one of the goals of his or her agenda from a cost/benefit perspective. The helper is to use empathic highlights, probing, and invitations to self-challenge to help his or her partner do this. Help your partner identify benefits and costs and do some kind of trade-off analysis such as the balance-sheet technique.
3. Help you partner clearly state the incentives and payoffs that enable her or him commit to the specified goals.

Example: Mai, a 28-year-old Chinese woman and a third-year doctoral student in clinical psychology, is discussing her commitment to her career goals with Steven, a fellow student. She is an only child and both parents and grandparents have been pressing her to get married and have children. She wants to establish herself in her career first. She has one more year to go in the program plus a year's internship.

MAI: If I don't get my degree and begin my career before getting married, I'll never finish. I know others can do this. But I would be feeling all sorts of pressure from family and friends.
STEVEN: So, from your perspective, it's almost now or never. But you're already under a lot of pressure. What about the cost-benefit equation?
MAI: I'm the first woman to break the mold in my extended family. So I have to expect some costs. I don't like hearing disappointment in the voices of my parents and grandparents. But I'm setting a direction for the rest of my life.
STEVEN: You're ready to pay the price. How do you counter the pressures?
MAI: First of all, I don't avoid them. I talk to them about how exciting I find my work. I talk to them about how this will benefit both me and whatever family I have in the future. Without saying it in these words, I ask them to be proud of me, not disappointed. I'm still the same daughter and granddaughter that they have always loved. I let them know by my actions that I love them. If I were to give in, that wouldn't be love. In my own way I let them know how *I* need to be loved.
STEVEN: What about social life? Any pressures there?
MAI: I have a couple of close men friends. But they know I'm not going to get into a very serious relationship right now. Eventually, I want someone who takes me as I am.
STEVEN: So there are a few bumps there, too.
MAI: None that I can't handle. I see myself as responsible and focused. If they want to see that as bullheadedness, well, that's their problem. Furthermore . . . .

And the dialogue continues in this vein.

143

4. After ten minutes of discussion, stop and receive feedback from the client and the person being helped. Use the video to debrief the session.

5. After the discussion, each member of the training group is to get a new partner, change roles, and repeat the process.

EXERCISE 12.10: COMPETING AGENDAS

When setting goals, clients often fail to see them in the context of the current range of demands on their time, energy, and resources. It is no wonder, then, that some goals do not get accomplished because they are squeezed out by all the other things clients have to do. In other words, clients have to face up to the reality of "competing agendas." Otherwise they end up trying to carry impossible burdens. Therefore, competing agendas need to be reviewed lest they block or dilute goals set during the helping process.

Example. Malik, 24 years old, is talking to members of his training group about a certain lack of progress in learning both the helping model and the skills that make it work. Now believing he knows what is happening, he says: "I came to this program all fired up to become the best counselor possible. But it hasn't quite happened. I know I'm not lazy. But this past week it struck me. I really enjoy the social life of this group. Lots of us have become friends. So much so, that my social life with the group has been doing two things. First, I'm letting it take up a lot of my time. I put off the work I should be doing. Second, I'm reluctant to challenge my friends in both group interactions and in one-to-one practice. This is being unfair to myself and unfair to you. I certainly want to enjoy the social life here, but I don't want it to compete with my original goal."

1. Look into two different goals you have set for yourself over the course of this training program.
2. Review the current commitments of your life both within the training group and outside. Outline the agendas that currently take up a great deal of your time, energy, and interest.
3. Indicate any competing agendas that might prevent you from accomplishing your goal.
4. Outline what needs to be done to manage competing agendas. This could mean dropping some current activities or reducing the scope of the goal.

Competing agendas for first goal.

_____

_____

_____

_____

_____

Ways of managing competing agendas.

_____

_____

_____

_____

_____

Competing agendas for second goal.

_____

_____

_____

_____

_____

Ways of managing competing agendas.

_____

_____

_____

_____

_____

Chapter 13

STAGE III:
PLANNING THE WAY FORWARD—
HELP CLIENTS DEVELOP PLANS TO ACCOMPLISH GOALS

Stage III is an important part of the helping process wherein clients find solutions and reach resolutions. Once clients are helped to establish goals, they often still need help to plan the actions or strategies that will enable them to accomplish their goals. These actions or strategies are solutions with a small 's'. Stage III has three tasks, all aimed at helping clients move to goal-accomplishing action.

Task III-A: Possible Strategies. Help clients brainstorm strategies for accomplishing their goals. "What kind of actions will help me get what I need and want?"

Task III-B: Best-Fit Strategies. Help clients choose strategies tailored to their preferences and resources. "What set of actions are best for me?"

Task III-C: Plans. Help clients formulate actionable plans. "What should my campaign for constructive change look like? What do I need to do first? Second? Third?"

Stage III adds the final pieces to a client's planning a program for constructive change. Stage III deals with the "game plan." However, these three "tasks" constitute *planning* for action and should not be confused with action itself. Without action, a program for constructive change is nothing more than a wish list.

TASK III-A:
HELP CLIENTS DEVELOP STRATEGIES
FOR ACCOMPLISHING THEIR GOALS:

There is usually more than one way to accomplish a goal. However, clients often focus on a single strategy or just a few. The task of the counselor in Task III-A is to help clients discover a number of different routes to goal accomplishment. Clients tend to choose a better strategy or set of strategies if they choose from among a number of possibilities. Read Chapter 13 before doing the exercises in this section.

EXERCISE 13.1: BRAINSTORMING ACTION STRATEGIES FOR YOUR OWN GOALS

Brainstorming is a technique you can use to help yourself and your clients move beyond constricted to imaginative or inventive thinking. Recall the rules of brainstorming but remember this one caution: Remain *focused* on the issue at hand; let your imagination roam freely but stay within the broad confines of the problem situation. Brainstorming is a technique. Use only if you think it fits the needs of the client. Don't force clients into using a technique that *you* think is useful but they see as foreign. That said, nudging is still a possibility.

- Encourage *focused* quantity. Deal with the quality of suggestions later.
- Do not criticize any suggestion. Merely record it.
- Combine suggestions to make new ones.
- Encourage even wild possibilities that stay focused on the problem situation. For instance, "One way to keep to my diet and lose weight is to have some part of my eating apparatus sewn up."
- When you feel you have said all you can say, put the list aside and come back to it later and add fresh ideas, but remain focused.

146

Example: Sam, a retired Caucasian lawyer in training to be a counselor, is in a high-risk category for a heart attack. Some of his relatives have died relatively early in life from heart attacks, he is overweight, he exercises very little, he is under a great deal of pressure in his job, and he smokes over a pack of cigarettes a day. One of his goals is to stop smoking within a month. With the help of a nurse practitioner friend, he comes up with the following list of strategies:

- just stop cold turkey.
- shame myself into it, "How can I be a helper if I engage in self-destructive practices such as smoking?"
- cut down, one less per day until zero is reached.
- use the new nicotine-based aids, such as patches and gum.
- look at movies of people dying with lung cancer.
- pray for help from God to quit.
- use those progressive filters which gradually squeeze all taste from cigarettes.
- switch to a brand that doesn't taste good.
- switch to a brand that is so heavy in tars and nicotine that even I see it as too much.
- smoke constantly until I can't stand it any more.
- let people know that I'm quitting.
- put an ad in the paper in which I commit myself to stopping.
- send a dollar for each cigarette smoked to a cause I don't believe in, for instance, the "other" political party.
- get hypnotized; through a variety of post-hypnotic suggestions have the craving for smoking lessened.
- pair smoking with painful electric shocks.
- take a pledge before my minister to stop smoking.
- join a group for professionals who want to stop smoking.
- visit the hospital and talk to people dying of lung cancer.
- if I buy cigarettes and have one or two, throw the rest away as soon as I come to my senses.
- hire someone to follow me around and make fun of me whenever I have a cigarette.
- have my hands put in casts so I can't hold a cigarette.
- don't allow myself to watch television on the days in which I have even one cigarette.
- reward myself with a weekend fishing trip once I have not smoked for two weeks.
- avoid friends who smoke.
- have a ceremony in which I ritually burn whatever cigarettes I have and commit myself to living without them.
- suck on hard candy made with one of the non-sugar sweeteners instead of smoking.
- give myself points each time I want to smoke a cigarette and don't; when I have saved up a number of points reward myself with some kind of "luxury."

Note that Sam includes a number of wild but focused possibilities in his brainstorming session. Now follow these steps.

1. On separate paper, develop two goals and then, by brainstorming, create a list of ways to achieve each of the goals. Add wilder possibilities at the end.
2. After you have finished your list, take one of the goals and the brainstorming list, sit down with a learning partner, and through dialogue expand your list. Follow the rules of brainstorming.
3. Switch roles. Through empathic highlights, probing, summarizing, and challenge, help your partner expand his or her list.
4. Keep both lists of brainstormed strategies. You will use them in a later exercise.

Goal # 1.

_____

_____

Goal #2.

_____

_____

EXERCISE 13.2: ACTION STRATEGIES—PUTTING YOURSELF IN THE CLIENT'S SHOES

Here are a number of cases in which the client has formulated a goal and needs help in determining how to accomplish it. You are asked to put yourself in the client's shoes and brainstorm action strategies that you yourself might think of using were you that particular client.

Example: Renalda, 53 years old, has been a very active person—career-wise, physically, socially, and intellectually. In fact, she has always prided herself on the balance she has been able to maintain in her life. However, an auto accident that was not her fault has left her a paraplegic. With the help of a counselor she has begun to manage the depression that almost inevitably follows such a tragedy. In the process of re-directing her life, she has set some goals. Since her job and her recreational activities involved a great deal of physical activity, a great deal of re-direction is called for.

One of her goals is to write a book called "The Book of Hope" about ordinary people who have creatively re-set their lives after some kind of tragedy. The book has two purposes. Since it would be partly autobiographical, it would be a kind of chronicle of her re-direction efforts. This will help her commit herself to some of the grueling rehabilitation work that is in store for her. Second, since the book would also be about others struggling with their own tragedies, these people will be models for her. Renalda has never published anything, so the "how" is more difficult. For her, writing the book is more important than publishing it. Anyway, these days self-publishing is always a legitimate option. Therefore, finding a publisher is not part of the "how." Here is one person's set of brainstormed possibilities for the "if I were Renalda" case.

- Get a book on writing and learn the basics.
- Start writing short bits on my own experience, anything that comes to mind.
- Read books written by those who conquered some kind of tragedy.
- Talk to the authors of these books.
- Find out what the pitfalls of writing are like, for instance, writer's block.
- Get a ghost writer who can translate my ideas into words.
- Write a number of very short, to-the-point pamphlets, and then turn them into a book.
- Do rough drafts of topics that interest me and let someone else put them into shape.
- Record discussions about my own experiences with the counselor, the rehabilitation professionals, and friends and then have these transcribed for editing.
- Interview people who have turned tragedies like mine around.
- Interview professionals and the relatives and friends of people involved in personal tragedies. Record their points of view.
- Through discussion with friends get a clear idea of what this book will be about.
- Find some way of making it a bit different from similar books. Brainstorm what I could do to give such a book a special slant.

Now do the same kind of work for each of the following cases.

Case 1. Emma, 27 years old, has been addicted to heroin. Her life has revolved around her habit. She has been told by her employer, an ad agency, that despite her creativity her erratic performance at work will

148

no longer be tolerated. She opts for a treatment known as ultrarapid opiate detoxification in which the drug naltrexone replaces heroin in the clients' opium receptors within six hours or so. Treatment with naltrexone is to continue for six months. Once she is free of opiates, her challenge is to build a very different lifestyle—one that will focus her talents and energies. She is in opportunity-development mode. This includes a new social life since, currently, she has no social life to speak of. One of her goals is reconciliation with her family, including her parents, one sister, and two brothers together with their families. She has seen very little of them over the past three years apart from attending two weddings. She wants to start the work on reconciliation while she is still feeling well. She realizes that reconciliation is a two-way street and that she cannot set goals for others.

Goal. If you were Emma, what would "reconciliation with my family" look like? If accomplished what would be in place? What would social life with the family look like? How is the goal conditioned by the fact that reconciliation is a two-way street?

_____

_____

_____

_____

_____

Brainstorming Strategies. What are some of the things you might do to achieve the kind of reconciliation with your family that you have outlined above? Do the focused brainstorming on a separate sheet of paper. Remember to include some "wild," but still focused, possibilities.

1. After you have developed your list, first share your goal with a learning partner. Give each other feedback on the quality of the goal. Note especially how you and your partner interpret "reconciliation."
2. Next share the lists of brainstormed possibilities. Working together, add several more possibilities to the combined lists.
3. Discuss with your partner what you have learned from this exercise.

Case 2. A priest was wrongfully accused of molesting a boy in his parish at a time when everyone who was suspected was considered guilty. Working with a counselor, he set three goals. His "now" goal was to maintain his equilibrium under stress. He knew that in the eyes of many he would be seen to be guilty until proved innocent. With the help of the counselor and some close friends, both lay and clerical, he kept his head above water. A near-term goal was to win the case in court. He also accomplished this goal. He was acquitted and all charges were dropped. After the trial the bishop wanted to send him to a different parish "to start fresh." He had been removed from his pastorate and was living at the seminary. But he wanted to return to the same parish and re-establish his relationship with his parishioners. After all, he had done nothing wrong. The bishop agreed to reinstate him in his parish.

Goal. If you were this man, what would "re-establishing my relationship with my parishioners" look like? What would be in place that is not now in place? Formulate a goal that has the characteristics of a viable goal outlined in Chapter 12.

_____

_____

_____

_____

_____

Brainstorming Strategies. What are some of the things you might do to re-establish your relationship with your parishioners, especially in view of the fact that some might still see you as tainted by the whole affair? Do the brainstorming on a separate sheet of paper. Include some "wild" possibilities.

Now, as in Case 1, complete steps 1-3.

EXERCISE 13.3: HELPING OTHERS DISCUSS OR BRAINSTORM STRATEGIES FOR ACTION

As a counselor, you can help your fellow trainees stimulate their imaginations to come up with creative ways of achieving their goals. In this exercise, use probes and challenges based on questions such as the following:

How: How can you get where you'd like to go? How many different ways are there to accomplish what you want to accomplish?
Who: Who can help you achieve your goal? What people can serve as resources for the accomplishment of this goal?
What: What resources both inside yourself and outside can help you accomplish your goals?
Where: What places can help you achieve your goal?
When: What times or what kind of timing can help you achieve your goal? What times might be better than others?

Example: What follows are bits and pieces of a counseling session in which Angie, the counselor trainee, is helping Meredith, a volunteer client, develop strategies to accomplish one of his goals. One of Meredith's problems is that he procrastinates a great deal. He feels that he needs to manage this problem in his own life if he is to help future clients move from inertia to action. Therefore, his "good intention" is to reduce the amount of procrastination in his life. In exploring his problem, he realizes that he puts off many of the assignments he receives in class. The result is that he is overloaded at the end of the semester, experiences a great deal of stress, does many of the tasks poorly, and receives lower grades than he is capable of. While his overall goal is to reduce the total amount of procrastination in his life, his immediate goal is to be up-to-date every week in all assignments for the counseling course in which he is enrolled. He also wants to finish the major paper for the course one full week before it is due. He chooses this course as his target because he finds it the most interesting and has many incentives for doing the work on time. He presents his list of the strategies he has brainstormed on his own to Angie. After they discussed the list, their conversation went something like this:

ANGIE: You said that you waste a lot of time. Tell me more about that.
MEREDITH: Well, I go to the library a lot to study. And I go with the best intentions. But I meet friends, we kid around, and time slips away. I guess the library is not the best place to study.
ANGIE: Does that suggest another strategy?

150

MEREDITH: Yeah, study someplace where none of my friends is around. But then I might not . . . .

ANGIE (interrupting): We'll evaluate this later. Right now let's just add it to the list.

(Then later in the dialogue.)

ANGIE: I know it's your job to manage your own problems, but I assume that you could get help from others and still stay in charge of yourself. Could anyone help you achieve your goal?

MEREDITH: I've been thinking about that. I have one friend. We make a bit of fun of him because he makes sure he gets everything done on time. He's not the smartest one of our group, but he gets good grades because he knows how to study. I'd like to pair up with him in some way, maybe even anticipate deadlines the way he does.

(Then later in the dialogue)

ANGIE: Your strategy list sounds good but a bit tame. Maybe it sounds wild to you because you're trying to change what you do.

MEREDITH: I guess I could get wilder. Hmmm. I could make a contract with my counseling prof to get the written assignments in early! That would be wild for me.

Note here that Angie uses probes based on the how, who, what, when, and where probes outlined above. She also uses the "wilder possibilities" probe. If you were Meredith, how would you react to Angie? Angie chose to use brainstorming. Critique how she did this. What other approach might she have taken? Share your thoughts with your two partners. Then move on to the exercise.

1. Divide up into groups of three: client, helper, and observer.
2. Decide in which order you will play these roles.
3. The client will briefly summarize a concern or problem and a specific goal which, if accomplished, will help him or her manage the problem or develop the unused opportunity more fully. Make sure that the client states the goal in such a way that it fulfills the criteria for a viable goal. Video the session.
4. Help the client discuss ways that he or she might go about achieving the goal. Use brainstorming only if the client seems to be stuck. If the client is stuck, give him or her a few minutes to write down a few possibilities. If the client does not seem to be stuck, do not use brainstorming. If you use brainstorming, explain what you are doing and why. Remember to keep the client in the driver's seat.
5. If the client is not stuck, simply help him or her discuss possible ways of achieving his or her goal. Use empathy, probes, and invitations to self-challenge to help the client move forward.
6. At the end of the session, stop and receive feedback from your client and the observer as to the helpfulness of your empathy, probes, and invitations to self-challenge. Use video in the debrief.
7. Switch roles and repeat the process until each has played all three roles.

TASK III-B:
HELP CLIENTS CHOOSE BEST-FIT STRATEGIES
"What Actions Are Best For Me?"

The principle is simple. Strategies for action chosen from a large pool of strategies tend to be more effective than those chosen from a small pool. However, if brainstorming is successful, clients are sometimes left with more possibilities than they can handle. Therefore, once clients have been helped to brainstorm a range of strategies, they might also need help in choosing the most useful. These exercises are designed to help you help clients choose "best-fit" strategies, that is, strategies that best fit the resources, style, circumstances, and motivation level of clients.

EXERCISE 13.4: USING CRITERIA TO CHOOSE BEST-FIT STRATEGIES

Just as there are criteria for crafting goals, so are there criteria for choosing best-fit strategies. The following questions can be asked especially when the client is having difficulty choosing from among a number of possibilities. These criteria complement rather than take the place of common sense.

Clarity. Is the strategy clear?
Relevance. Is it relevant to my problem situation and goal?
Realism. Is it realistic? Can I do it?
Appeal. Does it appeal to me?
Values. Is it consistent with my values?
Efficacy. Is it effective enough? Does it have bite? Will it get me there?

Example: Sam, the counselor trainee who wanted to quit smoking, considered the following possibility on his list: "Cut down gradually, that is, every other day eliminate one cigarette from the 30 I smoke daily. In two months, I would be free."

Clarity: "This strategy is very clear; I can actually see the number diminishing."
Relevance: "It leads inevitably to the elimination of my smoking habit, but only if I stick with it."
Realism: "I could probably pull this off. It would be like a game; that would keep me at it. But maybe too much like a game. But I know others who have done it."
Appeal: "Although I like the idea of easing into it, I'm quitting because I now am personally convinced that smoking is very dangerous for me. I should stop at once."
Values: "There is something in me that says that I should be able to quit cold turkey. That has more moral appeal to me. For me there's something phony about gradually cutting down."
Effectiveness: "The more I draw this action program out, the more likely I am to give it up. There are too many pitfalls spread out over a two-month period."

In summary, Sam says, "I now see that only strategies related to stopping cold turkey have bite. In fact, stopping is not the hard thing. Not taking smoking up again in the face of temptation, that's the real problem." The above criteria not only helped Sam eliminate all strategies related to a gradual reduction in smoking, but it helped him redefine his goal to "stopping and staying stopped." Sustainability is the real issue. He also noted that the brainstormed strategies he preferred referred not just to stopping but to sustainability. For instance, in the short term, the nicotine-flavored gum would reduce the craving once he has stopped.

1. Read the following case, put yourself in this woman's shoes, and, like Sam, use the criteria for determining the viability of the strategy she proposes.

Case: A young woman has been having disagreements with a male friend. Because he is not the kind of person she wants to marry, her goal is to establish a relationship with him that is less intimate, for instance, one without sexual relations. She knows that she can be friends with him but is not sure if he can be just a friend with her. She would rather not lose him as a friend. She also knows that he sees other women. She uses the above criteria to evaluate the following strategy: "I'll call a moratorium on our relationship. I'll tell him that I don't want to see him for four months. After that we will be in a better position to re-establish a different kind of relationship, if that's what we want."

2. Once you have done your analysis, share your findings with a learning partner. See what the two of you can learn from your differences.
3. Next review the reasoning that the woman herself went through and her decision. Here, then, is her analysis:

Clarity: "A moratorium is quite clear; it would mean stopping all communication for four months. It would be as if one of us were in Australia for four months. But no phone calls."

Relevance: "Since my goal is moving into a different kind of relationship with him, stepping back to let old ties and behaviors die a bit is essential. A moratorium is not the same as ending a relationship. It leaves the door open. But it does indicate that cutting the relationship off completely could ultimately be the best course."

Realism: "I can stop seeing him. I think I have the assertiveness to tell him exactly what I want and stick to my decision. Obviously I don't know how realistic he will think it is. He might see it as an easy way for me to brush him off. He might get angry and tell me to forget about it."

Appeal: "The moratorium appeals to me. It will be a relief not having to manage my relationship with him for a while."

Values: "There is something unilateral about this decision and I prefer to make decisions that affect another person collaboratively. On the other hand, I do not want to string him along, keeping his hopes up for a deeper relationship and even marriage."

Effectiveness: "When—and if, because it depends on him, too—we start seeing each other again, it will be much easier to determine whether any kind of meaningful relationship is possible. A moratorium will help determine things one way or another." Based on her analysis, she decides to propose the moratorium to her friend.

4. Discuss her reasoning with your learning partner. In what ways does your partner's analysis differ from yours? If you were her helper, how would you go about inviting her to challenge her reasoning and her decision?

EXERCISE 13.5: A PRELIMINARY SCAN OF BEST-FIT STRATEGIES FOR YOURSELF

You do not necessarily need sophisticated methodologies to come up with a package of strategies that will help you accomplish a goal. In this exercise you are asked to use your common sense to make a "first cut" on the strategies you brainstormed for yourself in Exercise 13.1.

1. Review the strategies you brainstormed for each of the goals in that exercise.
2. Star the strategies that make most sense to you. Just use common-sense judgment. Use the following example as a guideline.

- **Example**: Let's return to the case of Sam in Exercise 13.4. Remember that he is the counselor trainee who wants to stop smoking. Here are the strategies he brainstormed. The ones he chooses in a preliminary common-sense scan are marked with an asterisk (*) instead of a bullet (•).

*　　　just stop cold turkey.
*　　　shame myself into it, "How can I be a helper if I engage in self-destructive practices such as smoking?"
- cut down, one less per day until zero is reached.
*　　　use the new nicotine-based aids, like gum, advertised on TV.
- look at movies of people dying with lung cancer.
*　　　pray for help from God to quit.
- use those progressive filters which gradually squeeze all taste from cigarettes.
- switch to a brand that doesn't taste good.
- switch to a brand that is so heavy in tars and nicotine that even I see it as too much.
- smoke constantly until I can't stand it any more.
- let people know that I'm quitting.

153

- put an ad in the paper in which I commit myself to stopping.
- send a dollar for each cigarette smoked to a cause I don't believe in, for instance, the "other" political party.
- get hypnotized; through a variety of post-hypnotic suggestions have the craving for smoking lessened.
- pair smoking with painful electric shocks.
- take a pledge before my minister to stop smoking.
- join a group for professionals who want to stop smoking.
- visit the hospital and talk to people dying of lung cancer.
- if I buy cigarettes and have one or two, throw the rest away as soon as I come to my senses.
- hire someone to follow me around and make fun of me whenever I have a cigarette.
- have my hands put in casts so I can't hold a cigarette.
- don't allow myself to watch television on the days in which I have even one cigarette.

* reward myself with a weekend fishing trip once I have not smoked for two weeks.

- have a ceremony in which I ritually burn whatever cigarettes I have and commit myself to living without them.
- suck on hard candy made with one of the non-sugar sweeteners instead of smoking.

* give myself points each time I want to smoke a cigarette and refrain from doing so; when I have saved up a number of points reward myself with some kind of "luxury."

3. Share with a learning partner the Exercise 13.1 strategies you have starred (with an asterisk) for yourself and the reasons for choosing them. What makes each of the starred strategies "best-fit" for you? Have a critical conversation with your learning partner about your decisions.

4. Switch roles. Have your partner share his or her starred strategies and the reasons for them plus a critical conversation.

EXERCISE 13.6: BEST-FIT STRATEGIES—PUTTING YOURSELF IN THE CLIENT'S SHOES

In this exercise you are asked to put yourself in clients' shoes as they struggle to choose the strategies that will best enable them to accomplish their goals.

1. Review the case of Renalda in Exercise 13.2.
2. Review the strategies listed below that were brainstormed there.

- Get a book on writing and learn the basics.
- Start writing short bits on my own experience, anything that comes to mind.
- Read books written by those who conquered some kind of tragedy.
- Talk to the authors of these books.
- Find out what the pitfalls of writing are like, for instance, writer's block.
- Get a ghost writer who can translate my ideas into words.
- Write a number of very short, to-the-point pamphlets, and then turn them into a book.
- Learn how to use a word-processing program both as part of my physical rehabilitation program and as a way of jotting down and playing with ideas.
- Do rough drafts of topics that interest me and let someone else put them into shape.
- Record discussions about my own experiences with the counselor, the rehabilitation professionals, and friends and then have these transcribed for editing.
- Interview people who have turned tragedies like mine around.
- Interview professionals and the relatives and friends of people involved in personal tragedies. Record their points of view.

- Through discussion with friends get a clear idea of what this book will be about.
- Find some way of making it a bit different from similar books. What could I do that would give such a book a special slant?

3. If you have further strategies, add them to the list now.
4. Using your common sense, star the strategies you believe belong in the best-fit category.
5. Jot down the reasons for your choices. What makes them best-fit?
6. Share your choices and reasons with a learning partner and give each other feedback. Discuss what changes you would make to your choices.

EXERCISE 13.7: CHOOSING BEST-FIT STRATEGIES—THE BALANCE-SHEET METHOD

The balance sheet is another tool you can use to evaluate different program possibilities or courses of action. It is especially useful when the problem situation is serious and you are having difficulty rating different courses of action. Review the balance-sheet method in Chapter 13 of *The Skilled Helper*.

Example: Rev. Alex M. has gone through several agonizing months re-evaluating his career in the ministry. He finally decides that he wants to leave the ministry and get a secular job. His decision, though painful in coming, leaves him with a great deal of peace. He now wonders just how to go about this. One possibility, now that he has made his decision, is to leave immediately. However, since this is a serious choice, he wants to look at it from all angles. He uses the balance sheet to evaluate the strategy of leaving his position at his present church immediately. We will not present his entire analysis (indeed, each bit of the balance sheet need not be used). Here are some of his key findings:

Benefits for me: Now that I've made my decision to leave, it will be a relief to get away. I want to get away as quickly as possible.

- *Acceptability*: I have a right to think of my personal needs. I've spent years putting the needs of others and of the institution ahead of my own. I'm not saying that I regret this. Rather, this is now my season.
- *Unacceptability*: Leaving right away seems somewhat impulsive to me, meeting my own needs to be rid of a burden.

Costs for me: I don't have a job and I have practically no savings. I'll be in financial crisis.

- *Acceptability*: My frustration is so high that I'm willing to take some financial chances. Besides, I'm well educated and the job market is good.
- *Unacceptability*: I will have to forego some of the little luxuries of life for a while, but that's not really unacceptable. I know I can build some kind of satisfying career.

Benefits for significant others: The associate minister of the parish would finally be out from under the burden of these last months. I have been hard to live with. My parents will actually feel better because they know I've been pretty unhappy.

- *Acceptability*: My best bet is that the associate minister will be so relieved that he will not mind the extra work. Anyway, he's much better than I at getting people involved in the work of the congregation.
- *Unacceptability*: I can't think of any particular downside here.

Costs to significant others: This is the hard part. Many of the things I do in this church are not part of programs that have been embedded in the structure of the church. They depend on me personally. If I leave immediately, many of these programs will falter and perhaps die because I have failed to develop leaders from among the members of the congregation. There will be no transition period. The congregation can't count on the associate minister taking over, since he and I have not worked that closely on any of the programs in question.

- *Acceptability*: The members of the congregation need to become more self-sufficient. They should work for what they get instead of counting so heavily on their ministers.
- *Unacceptability*: Since I have not worked at developing lay leaders, I feel some responsibility for doing something to see to it that the programs do not die. Some of my deeper feelings say that it isn't fair to pick up and run.

Alex goes on to use this process to help him make a decision. He finally decides to stay an extra six months and spend time with potential leaders within the congregation. He will tell them his intentions and then help them take ownership of essential programs.

1. Choose a personal goal for which you have brainstormed strategies.
2. Choose a major strategy or course of action you would like to explore much more fully. If this exercise is to be meaningful, the problem area, the goal, and the strategy or course of action in question must have a good deal of substance to them. Using the balance-sheet methodology for a trivial issue would be a waste of time.
3. Identify the "significant others" and the "significant social settings" that would be affected by your choice.
4. Explore the possible course of action by using as much of the balance sheet as is necessary to help you make a sound decision.
5. Share your balance sheet with a learning partner. Through dialogue, give one another feedback and help one another improve the choices.

TASK III-C:
HELP CLIENTS FORMULATE VIABLE PLANS:
"What Kind of Plan Will Help Me Get What I Need And Want?"

A plan is a step-by-step procedure for accomplishing each goal of a change agenda. The strategies chosen in Task 2 often need to be organized and translated into a step-by-step plan. The plan should include only the kind of detail needed to drive action. Overly-detailed plans usually fall by the wayside. Clients are more likely to act if they know what they are going to do first, what second, what third, and so forth. Realistic time frames for each of the steps are also essential. The plan imposes the discipline clients need to get things done.

EXERCISE 13.8: DEVELOPING YOUR OWN ACTION PLAN

In this exercise you are asked to establish a workable plan to accomplish one of the goals you have set for yourself.

1. Choose a problem situation or undeveloped opportunity that you have been working on, that is, one that you have explored and for which you have developed goals and action strategies.
2. Indicate the goal you want to accomplish.
3. Write a simple plan that embodies the principles outlined in Chapter 13.

156

Example. Emma, a 27-year-old heroin addict who has just undergone an ultra-rapid opiate detoxification process and is now opiate-free, wants to establish or reestablish a social life that will include family and former friends. While on heroin, she either abandoned family and friends or they abandoned her. She has explored some ways of going about this with her counselor and settles on the following plan:

- She will contact a couple of friends and a couple of members of the family who she thinks might be most receptive to her overtures. She will first write them and tell them what has happened and what she wants to do. She will follow up with a phone call.
- Because she realizes that she might experience some rejection, she tells the members of her counseling group that she will need their support. Their support, both face-to-face and by phone, is an important part of her plan.
- When she is sure of the help of both a friend and of a family member, she will arrange to meet them separately face-to-face. She will use these encounters to get the "lie of the land" and to brainstorm further possibilities.
- She will use these initial reconciliations as a basis for further contacts. Hopefully her early contacts will also act as informal messengers to others within her family and among her former friends.

This is as far as she wants to go for the moment in the planning process. She will develop further plans only after a couple of successful contacts.

1. Before doing your own plan, get together with a learning partner and critique the plan that Emma has developed. What are its strong points? What are its deficiencies and how might they be remedied? What might you add to the plan?

The first goal you want to accomplish.

_____

_____

On a separate sheet of paper outline the major steps of your plan.

The second goal you want to accomplish.

_____

_____

On a separate sheet of paper outline the major steps of your plan.

EXERCISE 13.9: SHARING AND SHAPING PLANS

In this exercise you are asked to share and improve the plan you have developed and to help a learning partner do the same.

1. Share your written plans with a learning partner. Each of you should read the other's before you get together.
2. In a face-to-face session, explore and provide feedback to each other on the quality of each plan. How well shaped is it? To what degree is it simple without being simplistic? How concrete is it? What kind of compromise does it reach between too much and too little detail? How good is the fit between the plan and the person? Use empathic highlights, probes, and challenge to help the other shape his or her plan.
3. In the light of the feedback and dialogue, indicate what changes you would make in the plan.

157

The changes I would make in my first plan.

_____

_____

_____

_____

_____

The changes I would make in my second plan.

_____

_____

_____

_____

EXERCISE 13.10: FORMULATING PLANS FOR THE MAJOR STEPS OF A COMPLEX GOAL

If a goal is complex—for instance, changing careers or doing something about a deteriorating marriage—the plan to achieve it will often have a number of major steps. In this case a divide-and-conquer strategy is useful. That is, the complex goal—say, the improvement of the marriage—can be divided up into a number of sub goals. For instance, a more equitable division of household chores might be such a sub goal. It is one goal in the total "package" of goals that will constitute the improved marriage. In this exercise you are asked to spell out the action steps for two of the sub goals leading up to the accomplishment of some complex goal of your own. Consider this example.

Example: Bill, a clinical psychology student in a counselor training program, has discovered that he comes across as quite manipulative both to his instructors and to his classmates. He believes that he has developed the style as a response to the less than enthusiastic reception he received in past with peers, his parents, and previous instructors from his undergraduate program. His current style in working with others is to make the decisions himself while letting the other party think that he or she is having a say. Then, if he does not get his way, he moves to a more overtly domineering style. However, he realizes that this style is contrary to the values he wants to permeate his relationships, including, of course, his relationships with his future clients. Because this is the first time that he has received such feedback, one of the sub-goals he sets for himself is to get a very concrete understanding of his present style and to develop a better picture of a preferred style. This would be a major step in changing his overall manipulative style. Here are the steps in his plan to implement this style change:

- To elicit the cooperation of his instructor and the members of his training group. Bill wants to use the training experience as a lab for personal change.
- To spend three weeks interacting as he usually does. That is, for three weeks he will follow his instincts. He knows that he can't pull this off perfectly, because he is now observing himself more critically, as are the members of his group.
- To identify "live" instances when his domineering or manipulative style takes over. He can either catch himself or get immediate feedback from others when these instances take place. He will also keep track of instances of manipulative behavior in his everyday life.
- To identify "on the spot," but briefly, how the interchange with another person or the group might have gone better. This will provide him with a practical inventory of possibilities for a change in style.
- At the end of three weeks to draw up a portrait of the dysfunctional style and to pull together a portrait of the preferred style from the possibilities developed within the group.

1. With a learning partner evaluate the steps he has laid out. If he were to ask you for your help, what feedback would you give him about his plan? What changes might you suggest?
2. Now do the same for two of the major steps of a plan you have developed to achieve some complex goal related to becoming a more effective helper.

A key complex goal of mine.

_____

_____

One major step in the plan to accomplish this goal.

_____

_____

_____

_____

A brief description of the steps I would take to achieve this sub goal.

_____

_____

_____

_____

_____

_____

A second major step in the plan to accomplish this goal.

_____

_____

_____

_____

A brief description of the steps I would take to achieve this second sub goal.

_____

_____

_____

_____

_____

_____

3. Meet with a learning partner and share your plans.
4. Get and give feedback on the viability of the plans. What would you change?

EXERCISE 13.11: DEVELOPING THE RESOURCES NEEDED TO IMPLEMENT YOUR PLANS

Plans can be venturesome, but they must also be realistic. Most plans call for resources of one kind or another. In this exercise you are asked to review some of the goals you have established for yourself in previous exercises and the plans you have been formulating to implement these goals with a view to asking yourself, "What kind of resources do I need to develop to implement these plans?" For instance, you may lack the kinds of skills needed to implement a program. If this is a case, the required skills constitute the resources you need.

Goal. Indicate a goal you would like to implement in order to manage some problem situation or develop some opportunity. Consider the following example. Mark is trying to manage his physical well-being better. He has headaches that disrupt his life. "Frequency of headaches reduced" is one of his goals, a major step toward getting into better physical shape. "The severity of headaches reduced" is another.
Plan. Outline a plan to achieve this goal. The plan may call for resources you may not have or may not have as fully as you would like. Consider Mark once more. Relaxing both physically and psychologically at times of stress and especially when he feels the "aura" that indicates a headache is on its way is one strategy for achieving his goal. Discovering and using the latest drugs to help him control his kind of headache is another part of his plan.
Resources. Indicate the resources you need to develop to implement the plan. For instance, Mark needs the skills associated with relaxing. Furthermore, since he allows himself to become the victim of stressful thoughts, he also needs some kind of thought-control skills. He does not possess either set of skills. Finally, he needs a doctor with whom he can discuss the kind of headaches he gets and possible drugs available for helping control them.

160

Resources Plan. Summarize a plan that would enable you to develop some of the resources you need to move forward. In one program offered through the school, Mark learns the skills of systematic relaxation and skills related to controlling self-defeating thoughts. The Center for Student Services refers him to a doctor who specializes in headaches.

Problem situation #1: Your problem-managing or opportunity-developing goal.

_____

_____

_____

Skills or other resources such as social support you need to accomplish this goal.

_____

_____

_____

Summarize a plan that can help you develop or get the resources you need.

_____

_____

_____

_____

_____

Problem situation #2. Your problem-managing or opportunity-developing goal.

_____

_____

Skills or other resources such as social support you need to accomplish this goal.

_____

_____

_____

Summarize a plan that can help you develop or get the resources you need.

_____

_____

_____

_____

_____

_____

Share your goals and your resource-development plans with a learning partner and provide feedback to each other.

162

Chapter 14

IMPLEMENTATION: MAKING IT ALL HAPPEN

The Action Arrow of the helping framework indicates the difference between planning and action. Stages I, II, III and their nine tasks all revolve around planning for change, not change itself. However, the need to incorporate action into planning and planning into action has been emphasized throughout the book. That is, the "little actions" needed to get the change process moving right from the start have been noted and illustrated. We now take a more formal look at results-producing action. It is important to identify both the obstacles to action and ways to overcome these obstacles.

Stages I, II, and III are all planning stages. They are all just a lot of blah, blah, blah if the client does not engage in and persist in the kind of activity that accomplishes goals. Some clients, once they have a clear idea of what to do to handle a problem situation - whether or not they have a formal plan - go ahead and do it. They need little or nothing in terms of further support and challenge from their helpers. They either find the resources they need within themselves or get support and challenge from the significant others in the social settings of their lives. At the other end of the spectrum are clients who choose goals and come up with strategies for implementing them but who are, for whatever reason, stymied when it comes to action. Most clients fall between these two extremes. There are many reasons why clients fail to act on their own behalf:

- helpers who do not have an action mentality, who help clients discuss problems, but who do not help them act.
- client inertia, that is, clients fail to get started because change is hard work and there are obstacles in the way of constructive change.
- client entropy, that is, the tendency of clients to slow down and give up once they have started.

Often a failure to see serious down-the-road obstacles to action contributes to both inertia and entropy. Chapter 14, which deals with these and other implementation issues, should be read before doing the exercises below.

Since the skilled-helper framework is action-oriented, it is important for you to understand the place of "getting things done" in your own life. If you are to be a catalyst for problem-managing and opportunity-developing action on the part of clients, then reviewing your own track record in this regard is important. Unfortunately, helping often suffers from too much talking and not enough doing. Research shows that helpers are sometimes more interested in helping clients develop new insights than encouraging them to act on them. Inertia and procrastination plague most of us. The exercises in this section are designed to help you explore your own orientation toward action so that you may become a more effective stimulus to action for your clients.

EXERCISE 14.1: EXPLORING YOUR OWN TENDENCY TO PROCRASTINATE

Procrastination, putting things off, is part of the human condition. We all do it, at least sometimes. In fact, we can become quite inventive in procrastination. Some procrastination is chronic - "I never seem to get around to doing papers for my courses until the last minute." But procrastination can also be incident- or project-specific - "I know I promised to go see my ailing aunt who loves me dearly, but I haven't gotten around to doing it." In this exercise you are asked to explore either chronic or incident-specific procrastination in your own life.

An example of chronic procrastination: Dahlia, 52, whose children, including one autistic son, are now grown, has returned to school in order to become a counselor. She has this to say about her tendency to procrastinate. "My husband is in business for himself. I take care of a lot of the routine correspondence for the business and our household. Often I let it pile up. The more it piles up the more I hate to face it. On occasion, an important business letter gets lost in the shuffle. This annoys my husband a great deal. Then with a great deal of flurry, I do it all and for a while keep current. But then I slide back into my old ways. I also notice that when I let the mail pile up I waste a lot of time reading junk mail—catalogs of things I'm not going to buy, things I don't need. All of this is odd because now that I am in school time is at a premium and I need to become more efficient."

An example of incident-specific procrastination: Randolph, a 24-year-old counselor trainee, discusses a deferred reconciliation with a cousin who attended the same college and with whom he had a falling out in his senior year. He says, "In high school she had been the popular one. I was a late-bloomer, I suppose. I came to be very well-liked in college, while her social life was average. In senior year I found out that she had been telling lies about me behind my back. My success, I guess, galled her. I told her off and our relationship ended. It made family get-togethers difficult. We'd avoid each other, even though our families are close. So I found reasons to avoid family events. But I think we've both matured quite a bit over the last few years. I want to re-establish a relationship with her, but I keep finding reasons to put it off."

1. Describe an instance of chronic or project-specific procrastination in your own life.

_____

_____

_____

_____

_____

_____

2. What are the inhibitors? What keeps you from acting? What are the incentives for *not* acting?

_____

_____

_____

_____

3. What available incentives would help you move to action? What can you do to mobilize them?

_____

_____

_____

_____

_____

_____

4. Share your findings with a learning partner. What do you need to do to move beyond either your habit of procrastinating or the specific instance of procrastination you described?

EXERCISE 14.2: EXPLORING THE SELF-STARTER IN YOURSELF

While all of us have a tendency to put things off, we also have the possibility of becoming self-starters. Self-starters move to problem-managing and opportunity-developing action without being influenced, asked, or forced to do so. Skilled helpers are, ideally, self-starters. They have a sense of "agency" that enables them to help clients explore self-starting possibilities in themselves.

Example. Dahlia, whose chronic procrastination is described above, came up with the following list:

- "I never put off the things I like to do or think I am good at. For instance, I like the volunteer work I do at the hospital. No one has to put pressure on me to show up. Plus, I feel like I do a good job there. "
- "I make new friends easily. I don't wait for people to approach me. I take the initiative."
- "I plan family get-togethers and make them happen. Family solidarity is an important value for me. I do whatever I can to develop it."
- "I'm in no way a hypochondriac, but I do watch my health carefully. I get yearly check-ups, I see the dentist regularly, and if I experience symptoms that could mean something, I get myself checked out."

1. Describe four ways in which you are a self-starter.

_____

_____

_____

_____

_____

_____

_____

_____

_____

165

2. Describe two ways in which you would like to become a self-starter.

_____

_____

_____

_____

_____

_____

3. Share what you have learned about yourself as a self-starter with a learning partner. If you have trouble finding ways in which you are a self-starter or ways to become one, explore the implications of this with the training group.

EXERCISE 14.3: LEARNING FROM FAILURES

As suggested in the text, inertia and entropy dog all of us in our attempts to manage problem situations and develop unexploited opportunities. There is probably no human being who has not failed to carry through on some self-change project. This exercise assumes that we can learn from our failures.

Example: Miguel kept saying that he wanted to leave his father's business and strike out on his own, especially since he and his father had heated arguments over how the business should be run. He earned an MBA in night school and talked about becoming a consultant to small family-run businesses. A medium-sized consulting firm offered him a job. He accepted on the condition that he could finish up some work in the family business. But he always found "one more" project in the family business that needed his attention. All of this came out as part of his story, even though his main concern was the fact that his woman friend of five years had given him an ultimatum: marriage or forget about the relationship.

Finally, with the help of a counselor, Miguel makes two decisions: to take the job with the consulting firm and to agree to break off the relationship with his woman friend because he is still not seriously entertaining marriage as an immediate possibility. However, in the ensuing year Miguel never gets around to taking the new job. He keeps finding tasks to do in his father's company and keeps up his running battle with his father. Obviously both of them, father and son, were getting something out of this in some twisted way. As to his relationship with his woman friend, the two of them broke it off four different times during that year until she finally left him and got involved with another man.

Some of Miguel's learnings. Since Miguel and his counselor were not getting anywhere, they decided to break off their relationship for a while. However, when his woman friend definitively broke off their relationship, Miguel was in such pain that he asked to see the counselor again. The first thing the counselor did was to ask Miguel what he had learned from all that had happened, on the assumption that these learnings could form the basis of further efforts. Here are some of his learnings:

- "I hate making decisions that tie me down. If I say 'yes' to something, I am saying 'no' to everything else."
- "I pass myself off as an adventuresome, action-oriented person, but at root I prefer the status quo."
- "I am worried if I really have the skills necessary to be successful with the consulting company."

- "I am very ambiguous about facing the developmental tasks of an adult my age. I have liked living the life of a 17-year-old at age 30."
- "I enjoy the stimulation of the counseling sessions. I enjoy reviewing my life with another person and developing insights, but this process involves no real commitment to action on my part."
- "Not taking charge of my life and acting on goals has led to the pain I am now experiencing. In putting off the little painful actions that would have served the process of gradual growth, I have ended up in big pain. And I picture myself repeating the same pattern in the future."

Notice that Miguel's learnings are about himself, his problem situations, and his way of participating in the helping process. Now turn to your own life.

1. Recall some significant self-change project over the last few years that you abandoned in one way or another.
2. Picture as clearly as possible the forces at work that led to the project ending in failure, if not with a bang, then with a whimper.
3. In reviewing your failed efforts, jot down what you learned about yourself and the process of change.
4. Share your learnings with a learning partner. Help each other: (a) discover further lessons in the review of the failed project, and (b) discover what could have been done to keep the project going.

The self-change project that failed.

_____

_____

_____

Principal reasons for failure.

_____

_____

_____

_____

_____

_____

What you learned about yourself as an agent of change in your own life.

_____

_____

_____

_____

_____

What could have been done to keep the project going?

_____

_____

_____

_____

_____

EXERCISE 14.4: IDENTIFYING AND COPING WITH OBSTACLES TO ACTION

As suggested in an earlier exercise, "forewarned is forearmed" in the implementation of any plan. Identifying possible obstacles to a constructive change project is wisdom, not weakness.

1. Picture yourself trying to implement some action strategy or plan in order to accomplish a problem-managing goal. As in the example below, jot down what you actually see happening.
2. As you tell the story, describe the pitfalls or snags you see yourself encountering along the way. Some pitfalls involve inertia, that is, not starting some step of your plan; others involve entropy, that is, allowing the plan to run into a brick wall or fall apart over time.
3. Design some strategy to handle any significant snag or pitfall you identify.

Example: Jacob has a supervisor at work who, he feels, does not like him. He says that she gives him the worst jobs, asks him to put in overtime when he would rather go home, and talks to him in demeaning ways. In the problem exploration phase of counseling, he discovered that he probably reinforces her behavior by buckling under, by giving signs that he feels hurt but helpless, and by failing to challenge her in any direct way. He feels so miserable at work that he wants to do something about it. One option is to move to a different department, but to do so he must have the recommendation of his immediate supervisor. Another possibility is to quit and get a job elsewhere, but, since he likes the company, that would be a drastic option. A third possibility is to deal with his supervisor more directly. He sets goals related to this third option.

One major step in working out this overall problem situation is to seek out an interview with his supervisor and tell her, in a strong but nonpunitive way, his side of the story and how he feels about it. Whatever the outcome, his version of the story would be on record. The counselor asks him to imagine himself doing all of this. What snags does he run into? Here are some of them:

- "I see myself about to ask her for an appointment. I see myself hesitating to do so because she might answer me in a sarcastic way. Also, others are usually around and she might embarrass me and they will want to know what's going on, why I want to see her, and all that. I tell myself that I had better wait for a better time to ask."
- "I see myself sitting in her office. Instead of being firm and straightforward, I'm tongue-tied and apologetic. I forget some of the key points I want to make. I let her brush off some of my complaints and in general let her control the interaction."

How can he prepare himself to handle the obstacles or snags he sees in his first statement? Then what could he do about making sure he gets an appointment?

_____

_____

_____

_____

_____

How can he prepare himself to handle the pitfalls mentioned in his second statement? What could he do to deliver his messages in a decent but forceful way?

_____

_____

_____

_____

_____

Personal Situation # 1. Consider some plan or part of a plan you want to implement. In your mind's eye see yourself moving through the steps of the plan. What obstacles or snags do you encounter? Jot them down.

_____

_____

_____

_____

_____

Indicate how you might prepare yourself to handle a significant obstacle or pitfall and what you might do in the situation itself to handle it.

_____

_____

_____

_____

_____

_____

Personal Situation # 2. Consider some plan or part of a plan you want to implement. In your mind's eye see yourself moving through the steps of the plan. What obstacles or snags do you encounter? Jot them down.

_____

_____

_____

_____

_____

Indicate how you might prepare yourself to handle a significant obstacle or pitfall and what you might do in the situation itself to handle it.

_____

_____

_____

_____

_____

EXERCISE 14.5: IDENTIFYING FACILITATING FORCES

In this exercise you are asked to identify forces "in the field," that is, out there in clients' day-to-day lives that might help them implement strategies and plans, together with forces that might hinder them. The former are called "facilitating forces" and the latter "restraining forces."

Example: Sam, as we have seen earlier, wants to stop smoking. He has also expanded his goal from merely "stopping" to "staying stopped." He has formulated a step-by-step plan for doing so. Before taking the first step, he uses force-field analysis to identify facilitating and restraining forces in his everyday life.

Some of the facilitating forces identified by Sam:

- my own pride.
- the satisfaction of knowing I'm keeping a promise I've made to myself.
- the excitement of a new program, the very "newness" of it.
- the support and encouragement of my wife and my children.
- the support of two close friends who are also quitting.
- the good feeling of having that "gunk" out of my system.
- the money saved and put aside for more reasonable pleasures.
- the ability to jog without feeling I'm going to die.
- becoming more aware of the spiritual dimensions of life.

Now carry out the following tasks:

1. Review a goal or sub goal and the plan you have formulated to accomplish it.
2. Picture yourself "in the field" actually trying to implement the steps of the plan.
3. Identify the principal forces that are helping you reach your goal or sub goal.

Spell out a goal or sub goal you want to accomplish and they key steps you are taking to implement it.

_____

_____

_____

_____

Picture yourself in the process of implementing the plan formulated to achieve the goal. List the facilitating forces could help you to carry out the plan.

_____

_____

_____

_____

_____

_____

Which facilitating forces are most useful? What can you do to strengthen and use them? For instance, Sam focuses on three related facilitating forces: his pride, the satisfaction keeping commitments he makes, and feeling better by getting the "gunk" out of his system.

- Since he is a religious man, every morning he prayerfully recommits himself to his promise to quit.
- Every evening he congratulates himself for keeping his promises despite "flirtations with temptation."
- He periodically prides himself on becoming less dependent on chewing the gum that satisfies his craving for nicotine.
- He slowly and prudently increases his jogging time and "glories in the fresh air" in his lungs.

171

Now do the same for your action program.

_____

_____

_____

_____

_____

Finally, through dialogue, share your findings with a learning partner.

EXERCISE 14.6: DEALING WITH RESTRAINING FORCES

Now turn your attention to whatever restraining forces there might be "in the field." When these are weak, they can be brushed aside. However, when they are powerful, they must be dealt with. We return to the case of Sam.

Some of the restraining forces identified by Sam:

- the craving to smoke that I take with me everywhere.
- seeing other people smoke.
- danger times: when I get nervous, after meals, when I feel depressed and discouraged, when I sit and read the paper, when I have a cup of coffee, at night watching television.
- being offered cigarettes by friends.
- when the novelty of the program wears off (and that could be fairly soon).
- increased appetite for food and the possibility of putting on weight.
- my tendency to rationalize and offer great excuses for my failures.
- the fact that I've tried to stop smoking several times before and have never succeeded.

Now do the following tasks:

1. Review a goal or sub goal you identified in the previous exercise.
2. Once more, picture yourself "in the field" actually trying to implement the steps of the plan.
3. Identify the principal forces that are hindering you from reaching your goal or sub goal.

List the restraining forces that might keep you from carrying out the plan.

_____

_____

_____

_____

172

Which restraining forces are most powerful? What can you do to eliminate or minimize them? For example, Klaus is an alcoholic who wants to stop drinking. He joins Alcoholics Anonymous. During a meeting he is given the names and telephone numbers of two people whom he is told he may call at any time of the day or night if he feels he needs help. He sees this as a critical facilitating force—just knowing that help is around the corner when he needs it. However, Klaus sees being able to get help anytime as a kind of dependency. He hates dependency since he sees that its roots go deep inside him. This is a major restraining force. How does he handle it?

- First, he talks out the negative feelings he has about being dependent in this way with a counselor. That is, the first step in managing this restraining force is to name it.
- In talking, he soon realizes that calling others is a temporary form of dependency that is instrumental in achieving an important goal, developing a pattern of sobriety. He sees calling as a safety value, not a continuation of the dependency streak within him.
- Next he calls the telephone numbers a couple of times when he is not in trouble just to get the feel of doing so. He likes letting others know that he is in good shape.
- He puts the numbers in his wallet, he memorizes them, and he puts them on a piece a paper and carries them in a medical bracelet that tells people who might find him drunk that he is an alcoholic trying to overcome his problem. That is, he eliminates one excuse for not using the numbers.
- Finally, he calls the telephone numbers a couple of times when the craving for alcohol is high and his spirits are low. That is, he gets practice in using this temporary resource.

Now do the same for your change program.

_____

_____

_____

_____

_____

_____

_____

Finally, share your findings with a learning partner. Use empathy, probing, and challenge to help each other learn from the exercise.

RESILIENCE

Resilience refers to people's ability to "bounce back" from negative events in their lives. Often enough we read accounts of extraordinary resilience. But here we are talking about helping clients into the resilience that lies within most of us. Clients have to do it themselves, but therapists can help them. We start with your own experience of resilience.

EXERCISE 14.7: REVIEWING YOUR OWN RESILIENCE

Chapter 14 ends with a section on the importance of resilience. Getting in touch with your own resilience will help you spot resilience resources in your clients. Resilience means getting back on your feet after some kind of crisis or failure. It also means moving ahead in spite of continuing obstacles or opposition.

1. Think of a couple of instances of crisis or failure in your life that you handled well.
2. Describe what you did to get back on your feet.

Example. Nathan came back from a business trip to Southeast Asia extremely tired, with severe pains in his gut, and extreme diarrhea. Doctors first diagnosed diverticulitis and were considering surgery. Two days later they found that he had giardiasis. Bugs picked up during his travels were causing havoc in his gut. To make things worse the doctors were reluctant to give up the diverticulitis diagnosis and the surgical team kept circling him. Nathan was in the hospital for 10 days, an eternity in these days of managed care. The third day of his stay, he decided that he had to keep going. He put himself on a schedule. He got up at his usual time. He shaved. He put himself on a reading schedule. When he was too miserable to read, he walked the corridors endlessly dragging the intravenous feeding device along with him. He engaged the head of the surgical team in a discussion at the heart of which was this question: "If we know for sure that I have a bad case of giardiasis and if the symptoms of that disease are pretty much the same as a severe bout of *suspected* diverticulitis, why am I getting so much attention from the surgical team?" Nathan's motto was: "I'm not going to let this do me in physically and especially psychologically." He used the resources he used in his business life—a fighting spirit, lack of self-pity, self-discipline, logic, planning—to remain resilient in the face of the disease and medical fumbling.

Describe one crisis or failure that you feel you handled well.

_____

_____

Describe in some detail what you did to get back on your feet.

_____

_____

_____

_____

Describe a second crisis or failure that you feel you handled well.

_____

_____

Describe in some detail what you did to get back on your feet.

_____

_____

_____

_____

3. With a learning partner share answers to the question, "How resilient are you?"

EXERCISE 14.8: REVIEWING ANOTHER PERSON'S RESILIENCE

You have probably witnessed any number of examples of resilience among family, friends, acquaintances, work colleagues, fellow church members, and so forth. Not heroic resilience, but the kind of resilience many people are capable of.

1. Think of a couple of instances of substantial resilience you have witnessed.
2. Describe what these people did to get back on their feet.

Case #1.

_____

_____

In what ways did this person manifest his or her resilience?

_____

_____

_____

_____

Case #2.

_____

_____

In what ways did this person manifest his or her resilience?

_____

_____

_____

_____

3. What does this say about the possible resilience of clients you will be seeing? Share your thoughts with a learning partner.

EXERCISE 14.9: HELPING CLIENTS TAP INTO THEIR RESILIENCE

Encouraging resilience is part of the helping process. Although we draw upon our resilience, it is not a fixed trait—resilience can also be developed. Think of how you have been "toughened" by life's experiences and learned to bounce back when something did not turn out as expected—this is learning resilience. Review the section in Chapter 14 of *The Skilled Helper* that lists different possibilities for helping clients with this process, and then complete the exercise below. These areas can give you some ideas for helping clients identify ways to "tap into" and develop their ability to bounce back.

1. Read the imagined scenario below and answer the questions that follow the scenario (questions 1 and 2). The questions are designed to help you think about the scenario from both the client's and helper's perspective.
2. Get with a learning partner and role play (3-5 minutes), both taking turns as counselor and client. In the role of client, inject your personality and who you are into the role play, so as to give the role play "flavor" and to make it more genuine and real. In the role of counselor, use the counseling skills you have developed to understand what resiliencies the client has drawn upon in the past. Video the session.
3. Afterward, give feedback to each other from the client's perspective about what was helpful and what was not. Be specific in your feedback. Use the video to debrief the session.
4. Lastly, talk with one another about what it was like as the counselor to try and help tap into the client's resilience. What was easy about it? What was difficult? What did and didn't feel natural? How were your ways of drawing out one another's resiliencies similar and different?

Scenario:
Zalia has applied to medical school for the third time and just received the latest round of rejection letters. Her dream has always been to be a doctor and she is devastated. She has a parent who is a physician, and the rest of the family members (both immediate and extended) are all very successful in a variety of professional careers. Zalia is close to her family, but is ashamed at what they will think. She does not know what to do next and seeks counseling for help. During the first session, the therapist also learns that Zalia is an extremely hard worker, is well-respected and liked by teachers and peers, and is seen as someone who can be counted on. She is a good student but has struggled on the MCAT (medical school entrance exam), saying that she got "psyched out" the two times the exam was taken. The client considered physical therapy as a career but decided it was not "prestigious enough" to meet the family standard of success.

1. Therapist Perspective

Which factors revealed in the scenario might contribute to the client's resiliency?

_____

_____

_____

Which factors might stand in the way of drawing out the client's resiliencies?

_____

_____

_____

What kind of probes might be helpful to consider for identifying factors of resiliency?

_____

_____

_____

2. Client Perspective

Which factors would contribute to your resilience if you were faced with this scenario?

_____

_____

_____

What did you do to develop your ability to bounce back?

_____

_____

_____

_____

How could someone help you draw out your resilience to cope with this problem situation?

_____

_____

_____

EXERCISE 14.10: USING SUPPORTIVE AND CHALLENGING RELATIONSHIPS

Key people in the day-to-day lives of clients can play an important part in helping them stay on track as they move toward their goals. If part of a client's problem is that he or she is "out of community," then a parallel part of the helping process should be to help the client develop supportive human resources in his or her everyday life. In this exercise you are asked to look at strategies and plans from the viewpoint of these human resources. People can provide both support and challenge.

Example: Emily, a 40-year-old single woman, is trying to decide what she wants to do about a troubled relationship with a man. She knows that she no longer wants to tolerate the psychological abuse she has been getting from him, but she also fears the vacuum she will create by cutting the relationship off. She is, therefore, trying to develop some possibilities for a better relationship. She also realizes that ending the relationship might be the best option. Because of counseling, she has been much more assertive in the relationship. She now cuts off contact whenever he becomes abusive. That is, she is already engaging in a series of "little actions" that help her better manage her life and discover further possibilities. Over the course of two years, the counselor helps Emily develop human resources for both support and challenge.

177

- She moves from one-to-one counseling to group counseling with occasional one-to-one sessions. Group members provide a great deal of both support and challenge.
- She begins attending church. In the church she attends a 14-step program something like Alcoholics Anonymous.
- Through one of the church groups she meets and develops a friendship with a 50-year-old woman who has "seen a lot of life." This woman has Emily's permission to invite her to challenge herself whenever she begins feeling sorry for herself. She also introduces Emily to the world of art.
- Emily does some volunteer work at an AIDS center. The work challenges her and there is a great deal of camaraderie among the volunteers. It also takes her mind off herself.

Since one of Emily's problems is that she is "out of community," these human resources constitute part of the solution. All these contacts give her multiple opportunities to get back into community and both give and get support and challenge. Now move on to the following tasks:

1. Summarize some goal you are pursuing and the action plan you have developed to get you there.
2. Identify the human resources that are already part of that plan.
3. Indicate the ways in which people provide support for you as you implement your plan.
4. Indicate ways in which people challenge you to keep to your plan or even change it when appropriate.
5. What further support and challenge would help you stick to your program?
6. Indicate ways of tapping into or developing the people resources needed to provide that support and challenge.

Summarize your goal and action plan.

_____

_____

_____

_____

_____

Identify the human resources that are already part of that plan.

_____

_____

_____

Indicate the ways in which people provide *support* for you as you implement your plan.

_____

_____

_____

_____

_____

_____

Indicate ways in which people *challenge* you to keep to your plan or even change it when appropriate.

_____

_____

_____

_____

_____

What further support and challenge would help you stick to your program?

_____

_____

_____

_____

_____

Indicate ways of tapping into or developing the people resources needed to provide that support and challenge.

_____

_____

_____

_____

_____